A Primer on Musculoskeletal Examination

Evelyn D Sutton, MD, FRCPC

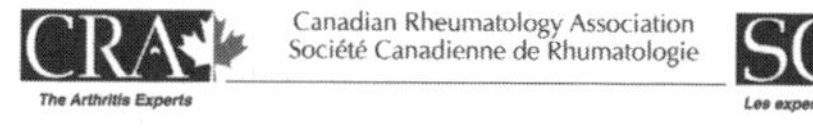

this title has received the endorsement of the Canadian Rheumatology Association

A Primer on Musculoskeletal Examination
Sutton, Evelyn D 1956 -

ISBN:	0-9688715-4-2
Editor:	Meagan B Louise
Techniques Model:	Jason Wong Brian Paul
Post-Production:	Duane Jones
Photography:	Rick Jemmett Jim Clark

Medical knowledge is updated regularly. As new information becomes available, changes to the assessment, treatment and management of various medical conditions are inevitable. The author and publisher have taken great care to ensure that the information presented is accurate, up-to-date and in keeping with the highest standard of professional practice at the time of publication. The author and publisher are not responsible for errors or omissions or for any consequences which may arise from application of the information in this book.

A Primer on Musculoskeletal Examination

Contents

Introduction		1
chapter one	Examination of the Hand	5
chapter two	Examination of the Wrist	11
chapter three	Examination of the Elbow	17
chapter four	Examination of the Shoulder	21
chapter five	Examination of the Cervical Spine	29
chapter six	Examination of the Lumbar Spine and Sacroiliac Joints	33
chapter seven	Examination of the Hip	39
chapter eight	Examination of the Knee	47
chapter nine	Examination of the Ankle	55
chapter ten	Examination of the Foot	59
chapter eleven	A Screening Exam	63
appendices	Selected Clinical Conditions; Normal AROM; Synovial Fluid Analysis; Glossary; Source Material & Suggested Readings	69
	About the Author	81

Dedication

To my father, Ray Sutton (1924-2006), whose optimism and enthusiasm for life and learning will always inspire me.

Acknowledgements

This book could not have been written without the overwhelming support of Dr. John Hanly, Division Chief of Rheumatology, Department of Medicine, Dalhousie University. His leadership and mentoring have fostered an atmosphere of collegiality and encouragement for research, clinical care and education. Dr. Hanly's view that medical education is to be valued, combined with his unwavering support of my role as a clinician-teacher, provided me with the confidence to write this book.

I am indebted to all the students whose enthusiasm for learning have inspired me to contribute as best I can to the learning process. Special thanks to my patients, some of whom are pictured in this book, who have agreed time and again to allow medical students and postgraduate trainees to practice their examination skills. For my colleagues and students who read the early drafts and provided their invaluable feedback, my sincerest appreciation.

For my husband, Rob, and children James and Ellen, thank you so much for your understanding and patience during all those weekend and evening hours when I had retreated to the computer room to work on this project. Thanks also to Jason Wong who, with patience and good humor, modeled for the anatomy and clinical photographs.

Last, but not least, a special thank you to Rick Jemmett - editor, publisher, photographer and friend - for his tireless efforts and unflagging enthusiasm for this project, without which this book would not exist.

ES

Introduction

History Taking Skills

In the first year of medical school, students are expected to begin developing the fundamentals of formulating a differential diagnosis, a potential list of causes that may explain a patient's symptoms. The first step in this process is obtaining a good history. A good clinical historian is a good listener, not passive but inquisitive, ensuring that all the pertinent facts and the chronological sequence of events are clear.

On initial presentation, many patients will complain about their 'arthritis'. This should never be taken at face value. Most patients mean they have joint pain, but not all arthralgias (the correct term for joint pain) are due to joint pathology. For example, shoulder pain may be the only symptom of a patient with ischemic heart disease. As in all fields of medicine, the history is the most important step in determining the cause of a patient's complaints while the physical examination helps to confirm or refute the diagnosis. The focus of this booklet is to aid the student in the physical examination of the peripheral and axial joints, but the examination must be done in the context of the patient's history.

One of the goals of the MSK interview is to determine whether the patient's symptoms originate within the joint or its associated tendons, ligaments or bursae, whether they are referred from a visceral or neurologic source, or whether the symptoms are due to a systemic inflammatory process. Questions pertinent to an MSK inquiry include the same questions one would ask of a potential cardiac patient presenting with chest pain:

- what is the **quality** of the pain?
- to where does it **radiate**?
- what makes it better? (**alleviating** features)
- what makes it worse? (**aggravating** features)
- what are the **associated features**?
- what are the **risk factors** for a particular cause of the symptoms? (including family history)

The MSK interview also includes additional questions of joint stiffness after periods of inactivity, in particular, the presence and duration of morning stiffness, and the impact of their symptoms on their 'activities of daily living' (ADLs for short).

The inquiry into functional losses is particularly important in the MSK inquiry. Losses may range from mild, where symptoms interfere with high demand activities such as sports, to severe, and impact on basic self care such as personal hygiene. For example, patients with severe losses of function may be reluctant to volunteer that they can no longer wipe their own bottoms; it is up to the clinician to explore the issues, which in turn allows for appropriate management.

While the onset of joint symptoms with trauma or a new physical activity is historically relevant, frequently the mechanism of injury is not so clear. In the absence of a reasonable injury mechanism, patients will frequently ascribe their symptoms to an activity which the physician can appreciate as being unlikely to have caused their problem. Alternatively, many patients will believe that they 'must' have sustained an injury despite having no recollection of any such event.

For example, if a young soccer player twists his ankle during a game and experiences instant pain, it is reasonable to suspect the trauma as the cause of his ankle pain. However, if he plays soccer and does not recall experiencing an injury, but nonetheless awakens the next morning (or even a few days later) with a swollen ankle, he may very likely claim to have somehow injured his ankle. This may be true, but in the absence of obvious trauma, it is also possible that his swollen ankle is the first manifestation of an inflammatory arthritis and the remainder of the history and physical examinations should be done with this in mind.

Sharp and severe joint pain is in keeping with acute joint swelling. The rapidity with which swelling develops in a joint correlates directly with the intensity of the pain. Trauma and the acute swelling of a gouty joint share this feature. However, gradual joint swelling typically manifests with less intense pain or 'soreness'. Pain in an arthritic joint is usually alleviated by rest and is aggravated with activity, but joint stiffness follows an opposite pattern. If pain accompanies only certain movements of the joint, it is likely that inflammation of a tendon or bursa is responsible for the symptoms. If any movement of the joint causes pain, the joint itself is most likely affected; if pain is present constantly and is made neither better nor worse with activity, consider a referred source for the pain.

Morning stiffness that persists for longer than 45 minutes is characteristic of inflammatory joint diseases such as rheumatoid arthritis. This is in contrast to the relatively brief duration of stiffness called 'gel phenomenon' experienced by patients with osteoarthritis. They too experience stiffness in their joints following periods of inactivity, but typically the stiffness eases within a few moments of using the affected joint.

A history of visible joint swelling, redness and pain should be sought. Recurrent attacks of joint pain and swelling with asymptomatic intervals may suggest a crystalline arthropathy such as gout or pseudogout. Also, the number and distribution of affected joints should be noted. Some diseases are characterized by the symmetry of joint involvement, others by their asymmetry.

Risk factors for inflammatory joint disease should be addressed. Just as the family history of early cardiac disease is critical information to obtain from the cardiac patient, a history of autoimmune diseases is similarly important in the MSK patient. A history of rheumatoid arthritis, systemic lupus erythematosus, psoriasis, inflammatory bowel disease or ankylosing spondylitis in a first degree relative of the patient should raise the clinician's index of suspicion of an inflammatory cause for the patient's complaints. Some infections can precipitate multiple joint swelling in the genetically predisposed host ('reactive arthritis'), and the history should include whether there has been any recent gastrointestinal or genitourinary tract infections.

Summary

A thorough and well-reasoned history will typically lead to the correct diagnosis; the physical examination is structured so as to confirm or reject the hypothesized diagnosis. When the history and physical examination do not support the same diagnosis, the clinician must think again. The history and physical examinations are dynamic, interactiveprocesses in which the clinician formulates and tests hypotheses regarding the cause of the patient's complaints, rejecting or accepting them on the basis of the information obtained.

Physical Examination Skills

In the following chapters, a basic screening examination of the peripheral and axial joints is described. Although each joint may have special tests unique to its particular anatomy or function, all can be assessed with a routine format which the student is encouraged to adopt. Each joint or region must be inspected for deformity, alignment, swelling, and redness. Bony landmarks, tissue temperature and crepitus are assessed on palpation. The movement of each joint is evaluated by checking active and passive range of motion. Common special tests for each joint are described, but the reader is encouraged to focus on the rationale behind the tests rather than committing them to memory.

Each section concludes with clinical vignettes to help apply the information, but confidence and proficiency can be achieved only through thoughtful practice. Therefore, the student is encouraged to practice their history and physical examination skills with every patient they see. If you enjoy problem solving, the MSK exam can be fun!

CHAPTER ONE

Examination of the Hand

A good deal of information about the patient's general health can be gleaned from the hand exam. The presence of clubbing of the nails, palmar erythema, splinter hemorrhages, peripheral cyanosis or asterixis should prompt the clinician to consider the potential associated conditions. For the purposes of this text however, common musculoskeletal conditions will be emphasized.

Inspection

No two parts of the body are easier to compare simultaneously than the hands. Look carefully at the palmar, dorsal, radial and ulnar aspects of both hands noting the colour and texture of the skin, the appearance of the nails, the alignment of the fingers and the bulk of the thenar and hypothenar muscles. It is surprisingly easy to miss rupture of the extensor tendons to the fourth and fifth fingers if one allows the patient to rest their hands in their lap, so be sure to view the unsupported hands. Nails should be inspected carefully for pitting; while one or two pitts are not significant, if several are seen then psoriasis and psoriatic arthritis may be present. Normally there is some scalloping between the flexed MCP joints; fullness may reflect synovial inflammation with effusions. Gnarled hands, frequently seen in the elderly, are from *Heberden's* and Bouchard's nodes, pathognomonic signs of osteoarthritis. Mallet finger, boutonniere and swan neck deformities should also be noted.

A summary of deformities you should be able to recognize (figures 1-5) includes:

- Heberden's nodes (DIP osteophytes)
- Bouchard's nodes (PIP osteophytes)
- Swan neck deformity
- Mallet finger
- Boutonniere deformity

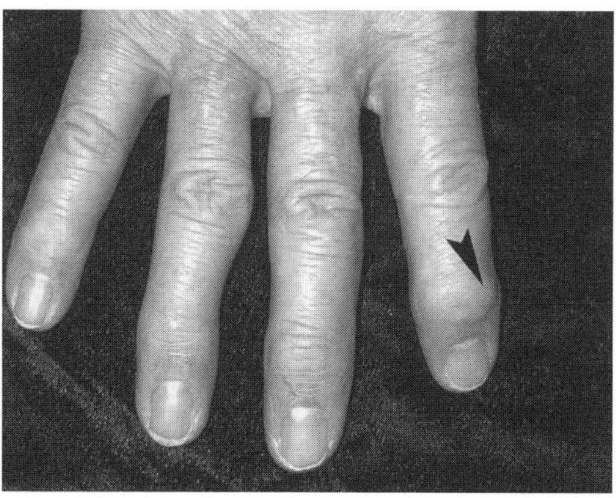

Figure 1. Heberden's nodes - most noticeable at the 2nd DIP (arrowhead) but also present at the other DIP joints.

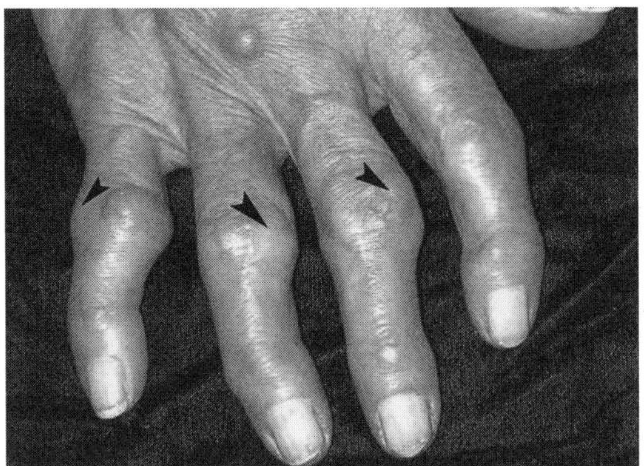

Figure 2. Bouchard's nodes.

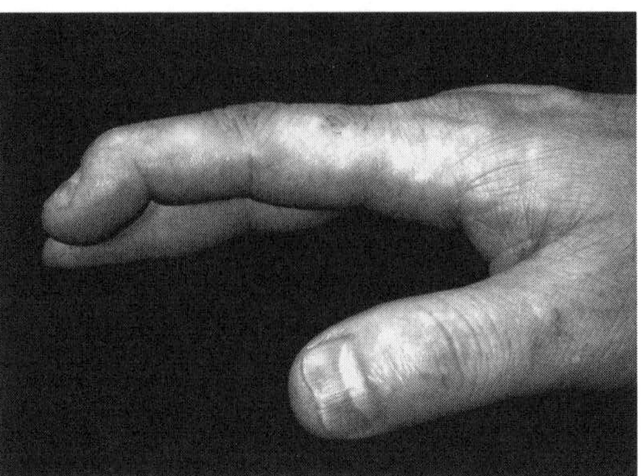

Figure 4. Mallet finger.

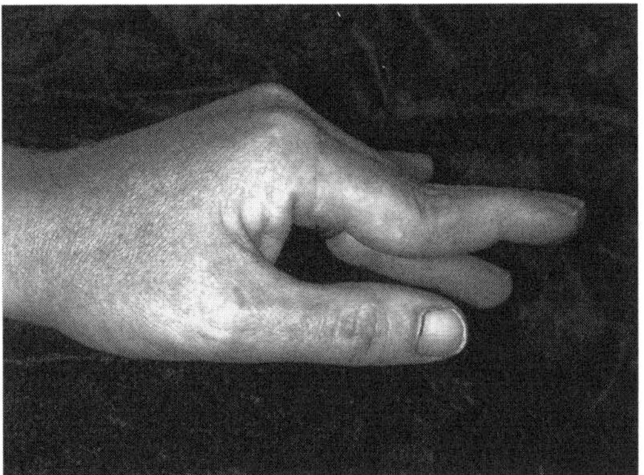

Figure 3. Swan neck deformity.

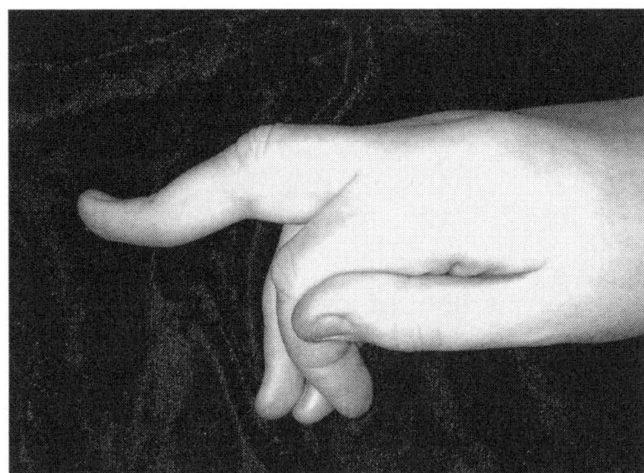

Figure 5. Boutonniere deformity.

Palpation

The skin is given close attention in the hand examination. Pick up a small amount of skin on the dorsal surface of the hand between your thumb and index finger and release it. Normally one will be able to stretch the skin only a few millimeters and the skin will fall back into place. Excessive laxity of skin may be indicative of an inherited disorder of skin and other connective tissues; one might therefore expect a generalized hypermobility of the joints (e.g. Ehlers Danlos syndrome). Conversely, a lack of elasticity and marked thickness of skin from injury or disease may result in loss of movement of the joints and secondary joint contractures.

Palpate all the finger joints for bony tenderness and/or enlargement and check each joint for effusion. Temperature testing is not reliable in the fingers as they are usually at ambient temperature. Start with the DIP joints and systematically examine each in turn, then move onto the PIP and the MCP joints. Do not forget to evaluate the thumb IP, MCP and CMC joints. Use a four-finger technique to evaluate for joint effusion (figure 6); lightly support each joint along its radial, ulnar, pal- mar and dorsal aspects (you'll need two hands). Apply pressure across the joint with two fingers and sense with the other two fingers whether any fluid is present.

Next check the palmar aspect of the hand

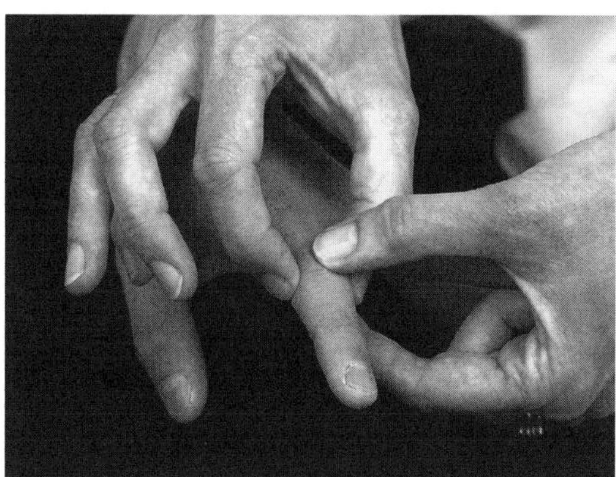

Figure 6. Assessment technique for finger joint effusion.

for signs of swelling in the flexor tendon sheaths and for contracture of the connective tissue in the palm (palmar fibrosis leading to *Dupuytren's contracture*). Palpate along the distal palmar crease for signs of tendon nodule formation and if the history includes finger locking or snapping, ask the patient to actively flex and extend their fingers to see if the locking can be reproduced.

Palpate the metacarpals in order. They are easiest to feel along their radial and dorsal aspects: keep your thumb on the palmar aspect and use your index and third finger to palpate along the length of the bones. Localized pain or interruption of bone may suggest a fracture.

Range of Motion

Do not be overwhelmed by the length of the upcoming list. Remember that there are a number of joints in the hand and each needs to be assessed, but with practice it can be done in a timely manner. The second through fifth fingers can be evaluated simultaneously and if no abnormalities are detected, individual testing is not required. The thumb is unique, however, and does need special attention.

Finger Movement (Figures 7-12)

- flexion and extension - MCP joints
- abduction and adduction - MCP joints
- flexion and extension - IP joints

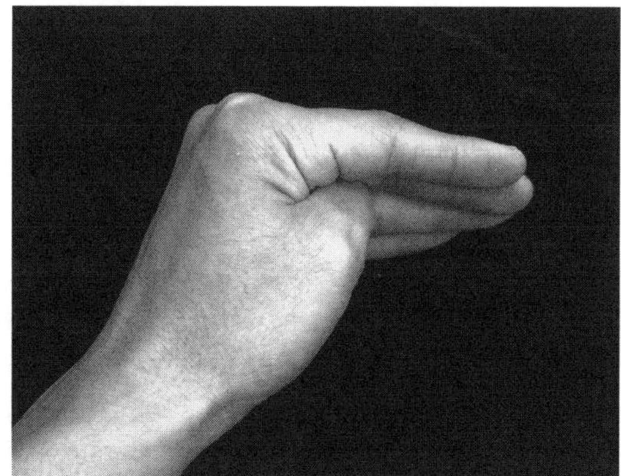

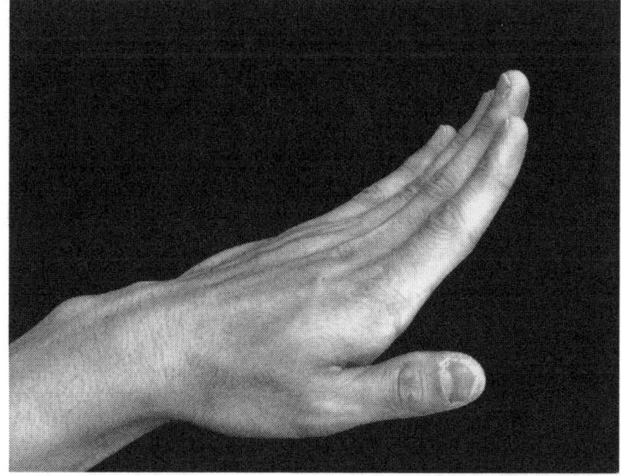

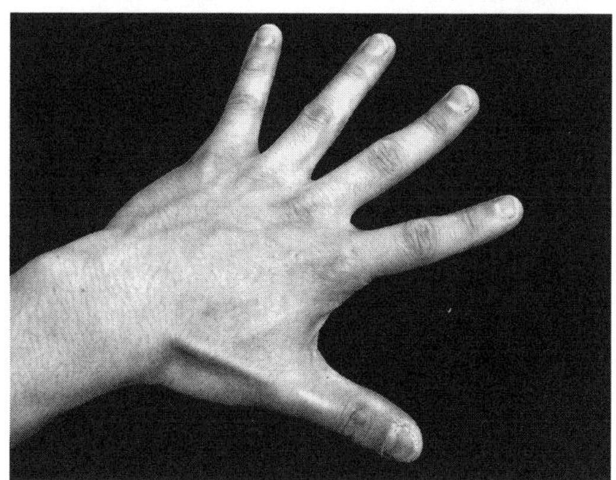

Figures 7 - 9. Top - MCP joint flexion. Middle - MCP joint extension. Bottom - MCP joint abduction.

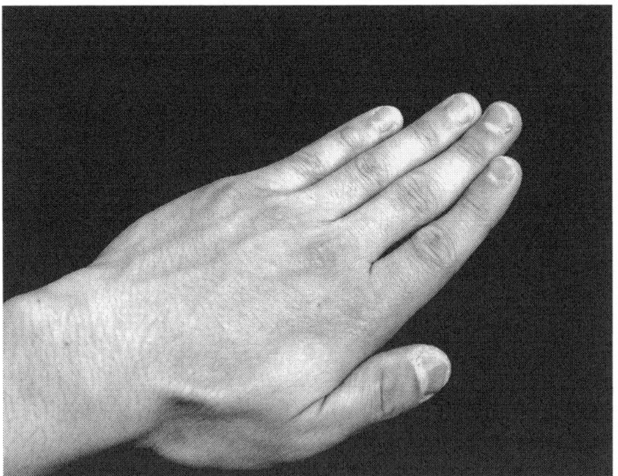

Figure 10. MCP joint adduction.

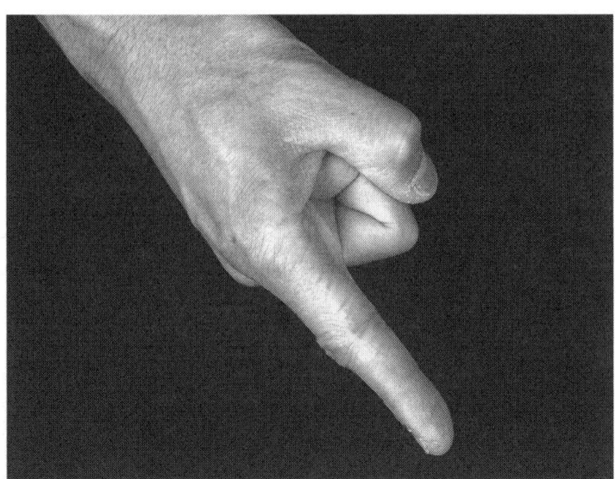

Figure 12. IP joint extension.

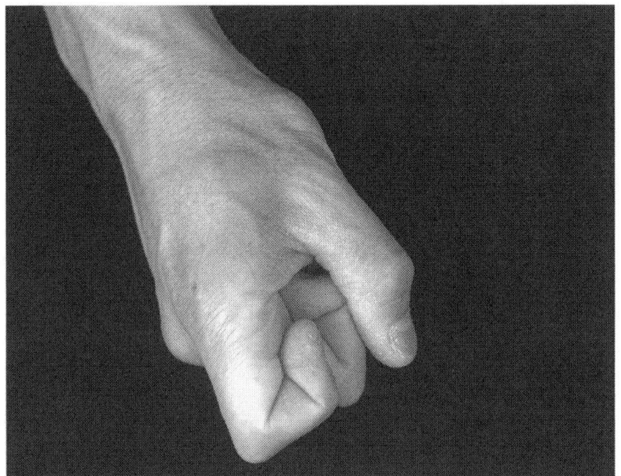

Figure 11. IP joint flexion.

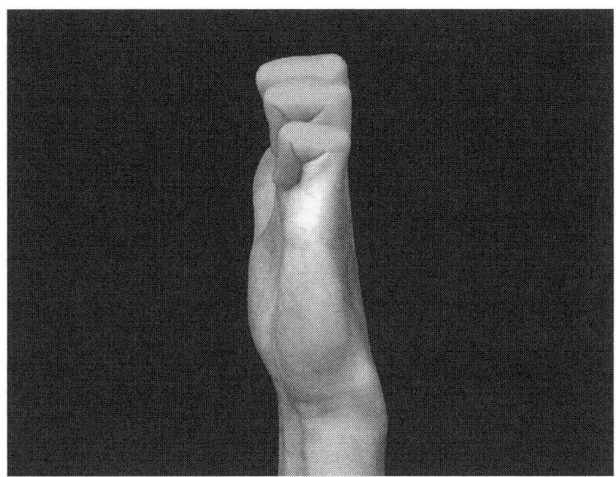

Figure 13. The 'Finger Tuck' Test.

A quick screening test for movements of the fingers is as follows. Ask the patient to make a fist (thumb out) and observe whether all the fingers can touch the palm. Then ask the patient to open their fist and tuck their fingers into a 'karate chop' or *finger-tuck* position, i.e. flexion of the DIP and PIP joints but extended MCP joints (figure 13).

Thumb movements.

To understand thumb movement nomenclature, look at your own thumbnail. Notice how it is oriented almost at right angles to the other fingers? This is the thumb's frontal plane. The thumb's MP and CMC joints abduct and adduct in a plane perpendicular to the palm, and flex and extend in plane parallel to the palm. (Figures 14-18). This is consistent with how we describe movement in the other finger joints: abduction and adduction occur around an antero-posterior axis, flexion and extension around a lateral axis.

Thumb Movements (Figures 14-18)

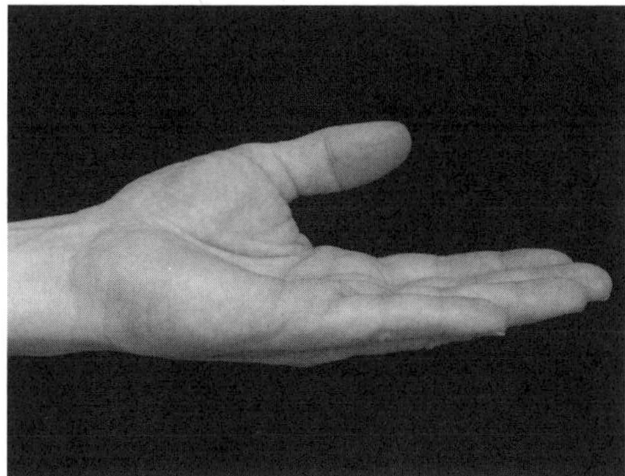

Figure 14. Thumb abduction

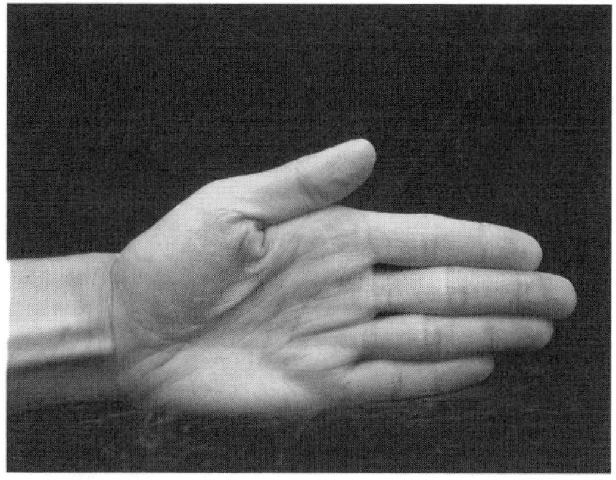

Figure 15. CMC adduction.

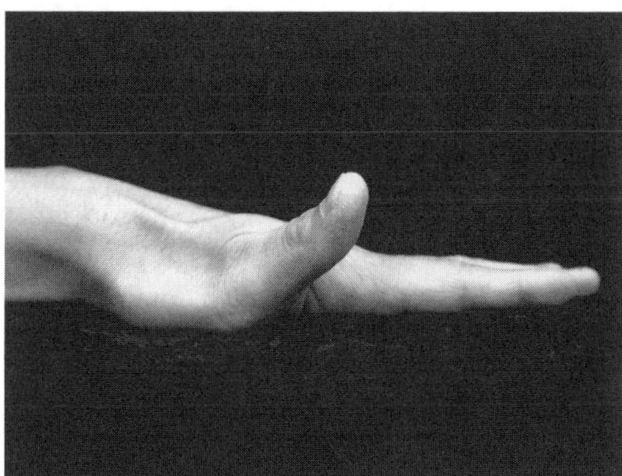

Figure 16. MCP joint extension.

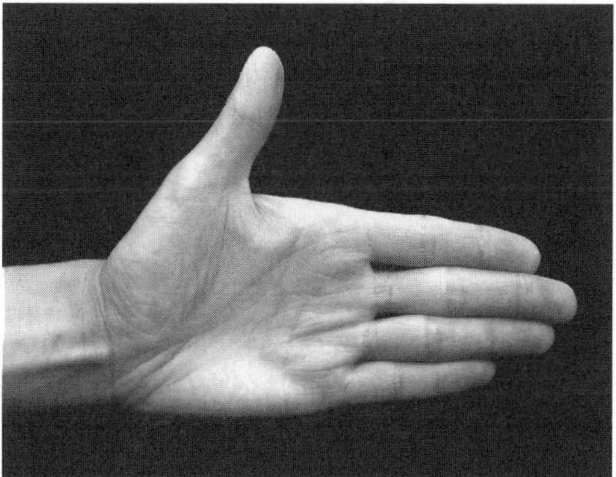

Figure 17. CMC radial abduction. (aka thumb extension)

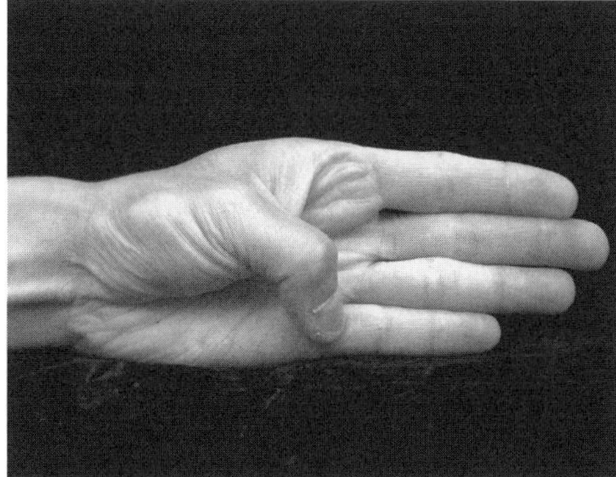

Figure 18. Opposition - (combined movement of CMC, MCP & IP joints

Clinical Vignettes

1. *A 35-year-old female homemaker presents with complaints of bilateral hand pain and stiffness. The second and third PIP joints in both hands have been the most symptomatic. The onset of her symptoms was insidious but dates to approximately six weeks ago. She is experiencing difficulty opening jars, turning doorknobs and doing up buttons. There is 30 minutes of morning stiffness. She has no other joint complaints.*

Even though the history is not complete, at this point you should already be forming a differential diagnosis. The insidious onset of symptoms and the presence of morning stiffness, although not overly long, are suggestive of inflammatory arthritis. The involvement of the PIP joints is not specific for inflammatory arthritis, however, and you should keep in mind the possibility of early onset osteoarthritis.

The physical examination is key to supporting or refuting your working diagnosis. Is there bony or soft tissue swelling of the tender joints? Is there restriction of movement actively and passively? If the exam is normal, be careful to label the patient with *arthralgias*, <u>not</u> arthritis.

If your exam does reveal soft tissue swelling of the precise finger joints the patient complains of, she definitely has arthritis. Further investigations would be needed. A woman of this age is at risk for rheumatoid arthritis, systemic lupus erythematosus, calcium pyrophospate deposition disease and, if there is a personal or family history of psoriasis, psoriatic arthritis. Referral to a rheumatologist would be appropriate. If your examination reveals bony enlargement of the PIP joints, osteoarthritis is the correct diagnosis and further investigations would not be required.

2. *A 26 year-old male letter carrier has noted painful swelling of his left ring and long finger DIP joints over the past 3 months. The joints have gotten very painful and red, and they never feel normal. Other joints have been painfree. He has had psoriasis since the age of thirteen, and is otherwise in good health. On examination there is redness and swelling of the left third and fourth DIP joints, and multliple fingernails are thickened and discolored. He has psoriatic lesions in his scalp.*

This young man has psoriatic arthritis. DIP involvement is almost always associated with psoriatic nail changes, so if they are absent, look for another cause. The peak age of onset for psoriatic arthritis is between the ages of 20-40 years.

CHAPTER TWO

Examination of the Wrist

Although the wrist is a complex joint with many bones and articulations, the examination need not be daunting. By following the basic principles of any joint exam the examiner can quickly evaluate the region and determine the cause of the patient's symptoms.

Inspection

Always inspect both wrists, looking for deformity, swelling, deviation or painful posturing. Remember to look from more than one view: dorsal, palmar, radial and ulnar. This can be quickly accomplished by having the patient hold their hands palms down, palms up, and with elbows flexed at 90 degrees and at 150 degrees. This is a good time to look for signs of extensor tendon rupture and/or a *tuck sign* in the rheumatoid patient. The tuck sign (bulking of the synovial tendon sheath with finger extension) is present in rheumatoid arthritis patients with proliferative synovitis of the common extensor tendon sheath. Have the patient make a fist (figure 19A) and then slowly extend their fingers (figure 19B). Look for this just distal to the dorsal wrist crease.

Clinical Hint:
In the absence of trauma, isolated swelling over the radial aspect of the wrist may be due to either tenosynovitis of the abductor and shortshort extensor of the thumb *(deQuervain's tenosynovitis)* or to osteoarthritis of the thumb's carpo-metocarpal joint. Swelling over the ulnar aspect of the wrist is very specific for inflammatory arthritis.

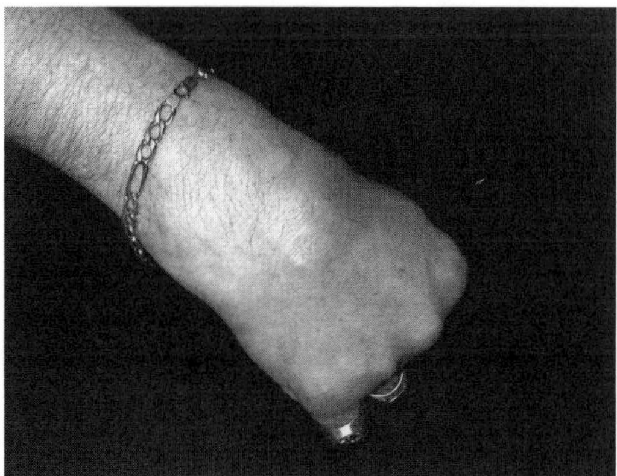

Figure 19A. proliferative synovitis, common extensor tendon sheath.

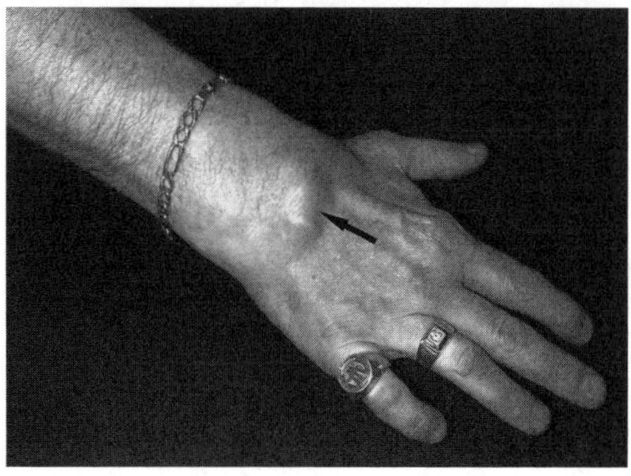

Figure 19B. the 'Tuck Sign'.

Untreated, tenosynovitis may lead to rupture of the common extensor tendons with loss of extension of the third, fourth and fifth fingers. Extension of the index finger is usually preserved because of its dual supply of extensors.

Palpation

Start first by checking for increased temperature in the joint. Use the ulnar or palmar aspect of your wrist to compare the temperature of the wrist to the muscle bellies of the extensor muscles and to the opposite wrist. Remember that the distal forearm is mostly tendinous and that the muscle bellies are closer to the elbow joint than the wrist joint.

Next, identify the important bony landmarks and note if tenderness is present:

- the distal radius and its tubercle
- the ulnar styloid
- the scaphoid (at the base of the anatomic snuff box - figure 20)
- the pisiform

Feel for soft tissue swelling. Normally there is an indentation just distal to the radial tubercle and at the base of the second and third metacarpals. When the wrist is swollen, full-ness will be appreciated. Palpate as well over the ulnar aspect of the wrist. You should be able to easily feel bone; if not, then prolifer- ative synovium may be the cause.

Range of Motion

Starting from the anatomic position, have the patient flex his/her elbows such that the palms face upwards. Evaluate all movements with the elbows flexed to eliminate potential contribution of movement from the shoulder. **From this position, evaluate flexion, extension, radial and ulnar deviation, pronation and supination.** You need not memorize specific degrees of movement, but one should be able to flex and extend approximately 90° in each direction. For supination and pronation the forearm should be able to rotate far enough to allow the palm to be parallel to the floor and ceiling (figures 21A and B).

If active range of motion (ROM) is restricted, you must move the patient's joint for them, i.e. passive range of motion. Be gentle and do the movements slowly, feeling for crepitus, clicking, or locking. Make note if the movement results in pain.

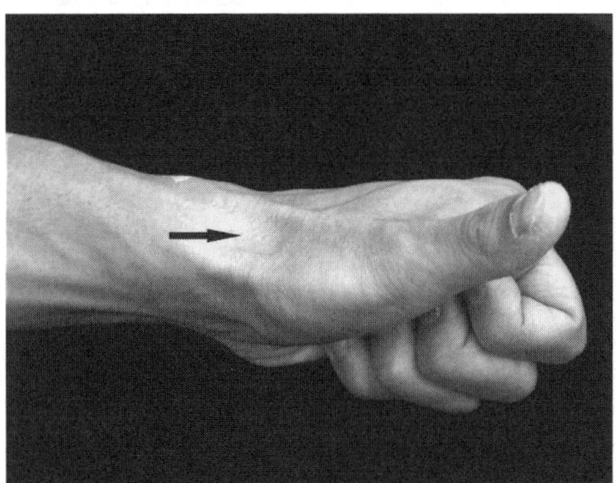

Figure 20. The anatomical 'snuff box' bordered by the tendons of the abductor pollicis longus & extensor pollicis brevis anteriorly & the extensor pollicis longus posteriorly.

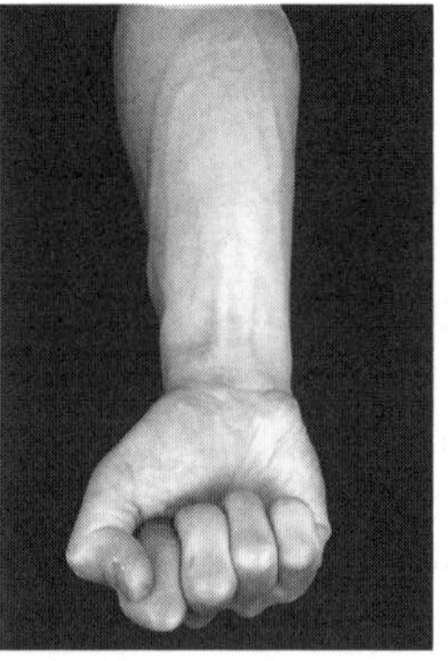

Figure 21A.
Forearm Supination

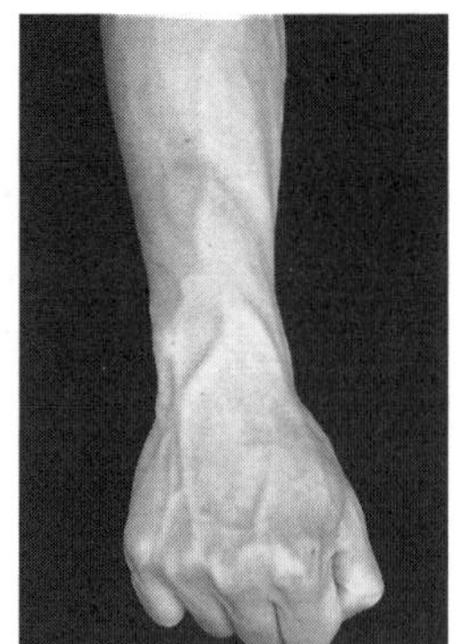

Figure 21B.
Forearm Pronation

Hint: can't remember which is supination vs. pronation? When the wrist is supinated it's easier for someone to put cash in your hand. When the wrist is pronated, money will pour out.

If passive ROM is normal while active ROM is decreased, weakness or guarding (voluntary or involuntary) may be the cause. If both active and passive ROM are similarly restricted, suspect a joint-based cause such as capsular adhesions, soft tissue contractures or end-stage joint disease.

Special Tests

Tinel's and Phalen's Tests are two standard tests for carpal tunnel syndrome, a common entrapment neuropathy of the median nerve of multiple etiologies. The theory behind *Tinel's test* is that if the nerve is compromised, it will be more sensitive to stimulation and pain will be produced in the distribution of the nerve. Thus, tapping along the course of the median nerve as it passes through the carpal tunnel may result in sharp, electric-like pain shooting into the palm, the fingers or up the forearm; such a response constitutes a positive Tinel's test. Note that mention is made of tapping along the *course* of the nerve; it is not adequate to tap only over the distal wrist crease, but rather a few centimeters above and below it, i.e., over the roof of the carpal tunnel (figure 22).

Phalen's test is equally simple. Flex the wrist, hold it in that position for at least a minute and ask the patient to report if there is any change in sensation in their fingers (figure 23). A positive test is attained when the patient reports numbness or tingling in the distribution of the median nerve.

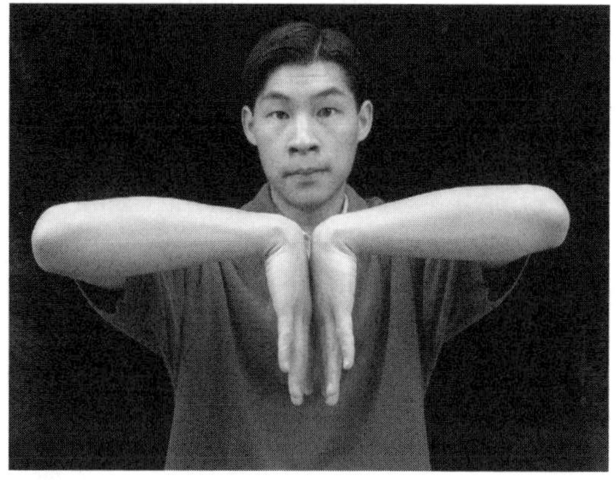

Figure 23. Phalen's Test.

Clinical Hint:
In a rush? Have three more consults to do before you go home? Have the patient sit with their hands on their hips, wrists flexed, while you check their head, neck and thyroid and/or auscultate their chest (figure 24). The time will go by more quickly for both of you. Phalen's test does not mean you have to have the patient sitting and concentrating only their hands.

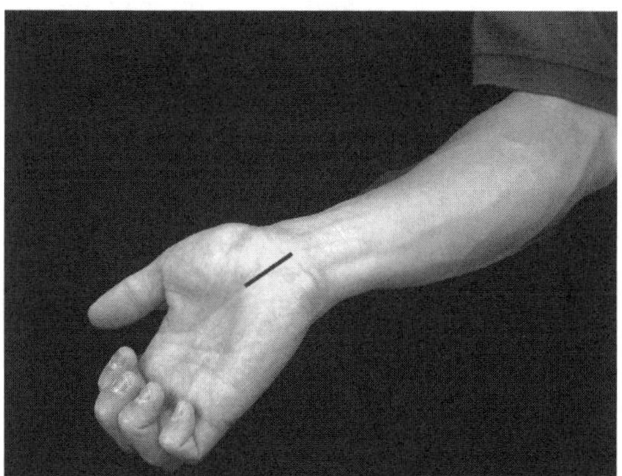

Figure 22. Tinel's Test - Median Nerve. Tap over length of tunnel, from entrance to exit.

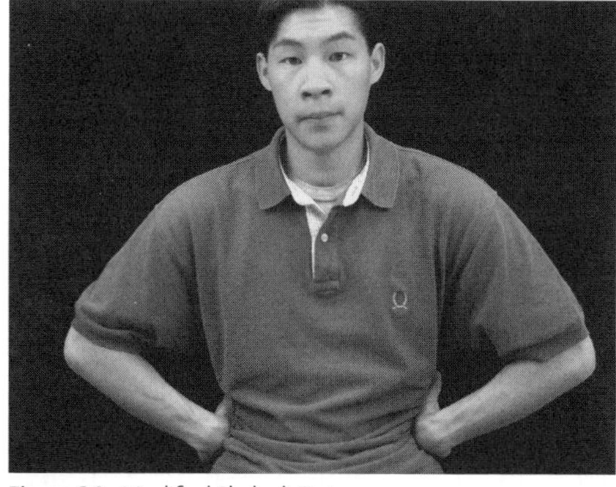

Figure 24. Modified Phalen's Test.

Finkelstein's Test: Pain over the radial aspect of the wrist? It's probably caused by either osteoarthritis of the thumb CMC joint or deQuervain's tenosynovitis, an inflammation of the lining of the sheath through which the abductor pollicus longus and extensor pollicus brevis tendons pass adjacent to the dorsolateral wrist. Remember the basic principle of testing for tendinitis: place the tendon(s) under a stretch or a stress. Finkelstein's test stretches the tendons. Ask the patient to tuck their thumb into their palm and move the wrist away from the radial side (ulnar deviation). If tendinitis is present this maneuver will elicit pain. You can confirm the finding by resisting radial deviation of the wrist. Note that other structures are stressed with this test, including skin, subcutaneous tissues, blood vessels and the superficial branch of the radial nerve. The correct diagnosis demands correlation of the history with the physical findings.

Other Tests: If you have extra time on the exam, you can test for strength of the wrist extensors and flexors. This also tests for lateral and medial epicondylitis. Tests for stability of the wrist are not usually expected from those not in a MSK related field of study.

Clinical Vignettes

1. *A 45-year-old male carpenter complains of pain and numbness in his right hand. He first noticed symptoms four to five months ago. Initially his symptoms were intermittent but lately the pain has been constant. It interferes with sleep and he has difficulties holding his tools because his fingers 'go to sleep'. The pain and numbness affect all his fingers. He has no other health complaints.*

At this point you should be very suspicious for entrapment of the median nerve at the wrist, frequently referred to as carpal tunnel syn-drome. The median nerve supplies sensation to the first three and a half fingers (thumb, index, long and radial half of the ring finger), so you might wonder why he has complaints of numbness in all his fingers. In fact, for many patients the intensity of the symptoms is so great that they do believe all of their fingers are involved. If the numbness is intermittent, you may be able to provoke the symptoms with Phalen's test, if so, ask them to concentrate and report if any of the fingers are spared. Usually they will be surprised to realize that at least one of their fingers is not involved. Remember to examine both upper extremities.

Although the most likely reason for his complaints is non-inflammatory narrowing of the carpal tunnel, look carefully for signs of swelling in the wrist and other joints. Phalen's and Tinel's tests should be performed, but even if these are positive, make sure to look for possible cervical nerve root compromise by testing the deep tendon reflexes.

2. *A 40-year old female radiologist presents with a chief complaint of left wrist pain of acute onset four days ago. Pain is sharp and located over the radial aspect of the wrist. She has difficulty turning doorknobs and picking up her briefcase. She is right handed so has been able to cope, but she is very concerned as she has noted swelling over the radial aspect of her wrist and there is a family history of rheumatoid arthritis. She has not been engaged in strenuous or repetitive activities, and can think of no reason why her wrist is sore.*

On examination, there is swelling over the radial aspect of the left wrist, and there is pain with both active and passive ulnar deviation of the wrist. Finkelstein's test is positive. A detailed examination of other joints is completely normal.

This woman clearly has deQuervain's tenosynovitis. The findings prompted a more detailed history. She had not been painting, doing yard or housework which may have set her up for the problem, but after closer questioning she did recall that the day prior to the onset of her symptoms she had used her left hand rather than her right to dictate reports for over 100 radiographs. She had held the tape recorder in her left hand and repetitively flexed and extended the left thumb IP, MCP and CMC joints, straining not the joints but the extensor pollicus brevis tendon. She had not recognized this as the potential cause for her discomfort, but the moment she tried to use her left hand to simulate the motion of using the tape recorder, the pain immediately recurred. Ice, rest and avoidance of using her left hand to dictate resolved the problem.

Many patients are fearful of the worst, and cannot honestly recall a precipitating event. Other patients ascribe symptoms to an event which may be totally innocent in precipitating their symptoms. Your job as the clinician is to weigh the evidence and decide whether to discard the information or to search for more.

CHAPTER THREE

Examination of the Elbow

Inspection

A sore elbow is usually held in a semi-flexed position, a posture that may become permanent if the cause of the pain is not dealt with in a timely fashion. It is easiest to inspect the elbows if the patient stands with their arms hanging at their sides, palms facing forwards (the so-called 'anatomic position').

First, observe the carrying angle of the elbow. (figure 25). If you could draw a straight line from the mid-shaft of the humerus to the midpoint of the distal wrist crease, the angle would be zero. Normally the angle is between 0 and 15° valgus but it may be as high as 20° in women.

Any degree of varus angulation is abnormaland should be noted. Remember to look from the side to detect either a flexion contracture or hyperextension, and view the posterior aspect of the elbow for olecranon bursal swelling or nodule formation. Swelling in the elbow joint is most easily seen as a fullness in the lateral infracondylar recess.

Palpation

Important bony landmarks at the elbow are:

- medial epicondyle (ME - figure 26)
- lateral epicondyle (LE - figure 26)
- olecranon tip (O - figures 26 & 27)
- radial head (R - figure 27)

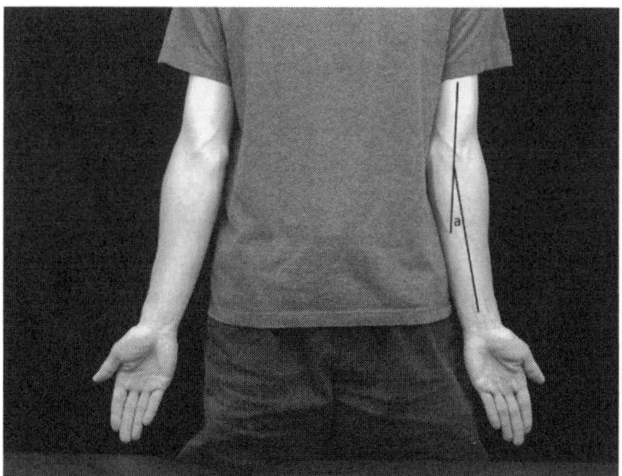

Figure 25. 'a' represents the carrying angle of the elbow

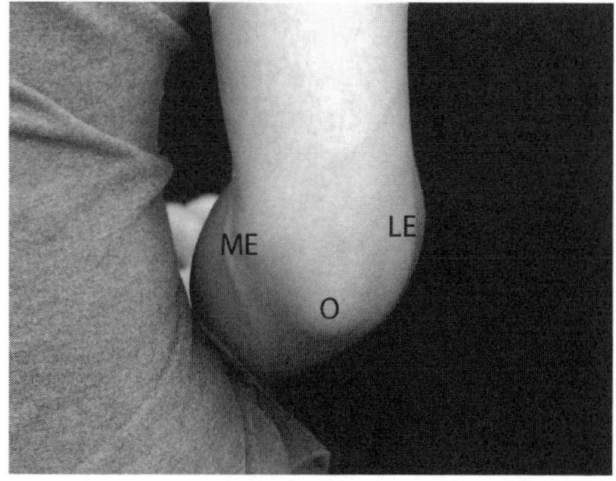

Figure 26. Bony landmarks - Elbow

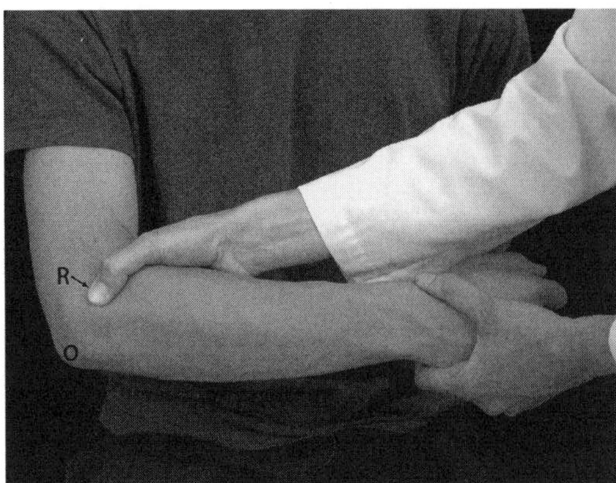

Figure 27: Palpation of the head of the radius

Clinical Hint:
Palpation of the radial head is easiest with the elbow at 90°. Identify the lateral epicondyle, then move your fingers just a few centimeters distally and ask the patient to pronate and supinate their forearm (figure 27). You should be able to feel the radial head rolling under your fingertips.

The important soft tissue landmarks of the elbow region are: the olecranon bursa, the ulnar nerve, and any nodules that might be present.

An elbow effusion is most easily appreciated in the lateral infracondylar recess with the elbow flexed at 90°.

Range of Motion

The movements available at the elbow are: flexion, extension, pronation and supination.

Assess these movements actively; if restricted, perform them passively. Normally, flexion and extension ranges between 0 and 150°, but one can remain functional with a minimum of 30-130°. Pronation and supination must be assessed with the elbow flexed; otherwise, you risk measuring internal and external rotation of the glenohumeral joint. Full supination and pronation allows the palm to be parallel with the floor and ceiling.

Special Tests

Tinel's test is not restricted to the wrist. Any nerve that is near the skin surface can be tapped to assess irritability. At the elbow the ulnar nerve is frequently inadvertently hit (as in striking one's 'funny bone'). If you think back to your own personal experience you will realize that accidental hits occur when the elbow is flexed; when the elbow is extended, the nerve is relatively protected. Thus, to perform Tinel's test at the elbow, flex the patient's elbow and tap over the ulnar nerve as it courses in the medial infracondylar groove. Tests for elbow stability are not usually expected from those not in a MSK-related field of study.

Resisted testing at the elbow may help differentiate between articular and musculotendinous sources of pain. Pain that is present with resisted movement but is absent with passive movement suggests a musculotendinous cause. Pain with passive movement suggests intra-articular pathology.

Golfer's Elbow - Medial Epicondylitis

Test by stretching or stressing the tendinous attachments of the wrist flexors. Stretch the attachments by supinating the patient's forearm while extending the wrist and elbow. Stress the tendons by resisting wrist flexion. This test will cause pain at the inner (ulnar) side of the elbow but it does not radiate far, rarely beyond the mid-forearm.

Tennis Elbow - Lateral Epicondylitis

Test by stretching or stressing the tendinous attachments of the extensor carpi radialis brevis and longus muscles at the lateral epicondyle of the elbow. Stretch the tendons by flexing the wrist, pronating the forearm and extending the elbow. Stress the tendinous attachments by resisting wrist extension. These tests are considered positive if they elicit pain over the lateral aspect of the elbow, with radiation to the dorsum of the forearm and occasionally as far as the dorsum of the hand.

Clinical Hint:
True tendonitis should respond promptly and completely to appropriate treatment. Failure to respond should prompt the clinician to reconsider the diagnosis.

Complaints of pain but a normal elbow exam? Remember to examine the joint above and below and do neurologic testing, including tests of motor strength, sensation and reflexes.

Clinical Vignettes

1. *A 55-year-old banker presents with a chief complaint of pain, swelling and redness of his left elbow. He has never had joint pains before and he has enjoyed good general health all his life. He first noticed discomfort in his elbow yesterday afternoon, but overnight the pain has worsened and the elbow feels hot to him.*

On examination there is marked redness and swelling over the dorsal aspect of the elbow and the extensor surface of the elbow is hot to touch. He has full extension of the elbow and there is no restriction of supination or pronation, but on flexion pain is increased and you note the swelling becomes more visibly prominent. The swelling is well circumscribed and the extensor surface of the elbow looks as if there was a small red tennis ball under the skin. What is the diagnosis?

First you must decide whether the problem is extra-articular or intra-articular. The fact that the patient can supinate and pronate the forearm without pain strongly points away from a process within the joint. In addition, if the elbow joint proper was swollen, there would be restriction of elbow extension as well as flexion. The swelling is located in the region of the olecranon bursa and the diagnosis is olecranon bursitis. The bursa must be drained and the fluid sent for the "three C's": Cells, Crystal and Culture. In the absence of a his- tory of gout, this patient should be treated with antibiotics while you await the lab results.

The olecranon bursa is a frequent site for infection, probably because it is prone to abrasions. Fortunately, there is no communication between the bursa and the elbow joint, so septic arthritis is not a usual sequela of septic bursitis.

2. *A 72-year-old retired locomotive engineer complains of pain over the lateral aspect of his right elbow. It has been present intermittently for the past 4 months but lately it has been getting worse. He cannot relate it to activity. Nothing seems to make it better or worse. There are no associated features. His general health has been good.*

On examination, inspection, palpation and range of motion of the elbow are within normal limits. Resisted wrist extension does cause some lateral elbow tenderness, but it is mild and is not identical to his 'typical' pain. What is the diagnosis?

At this point, one cannot form a diagnosis, although the problem does not appear to be originating from within or around the elbow joint. Do not be fooled by one weakly positive test for lateral epicondylitis. In this circumstance the history is not in keeping with the disorder and the exam findings are by no means diagnostic. In this scenario, you should be very suspicious of referred pain originating in the shoulder, or more likely, the neck. A careful examination of the cervical spine including deep tendon reflexes should be performed.

CHAPTER FOUR

Examination of the Shoulder

Inspection

The examination of the shoulder, like that of any other region or system, begins with inspection. Observe the movement of the arms when the patient is walking and when they remove their jacket or shirt. Fluid movement of the shoulder will be observed in the healthy shoulder as the patient walks and disrobes. Jerky, cautious or hesitant movements suggest pain or an adaptive response to mechanical problems within or surrounding the shoulder region.

Both shoulder regions should be inspected simultaneously, looking for effusions and asymmetry of muscle bulk, abnormal postures or bony irregularities. Subtle effusions are best appreciated as a loss of the normal deltopectoral groove (figure 28A). Wasting of the supra- spinatus muscle will be present in almost any chronic condition affecting the shoulder, including simple disuse atrophy, rotator cuff tendinitis, glenohumeral disease and a C4/5 or C5/6 radiculopathy. The shoulder should be inspected from more than one perspective. Do not forget to look posteriorly for winging of the scapulae. The clavicle is covered by little other than skin, and bony irregularities are usually easily appreciated.

Palpation

The glenohumeral joint is deep and an increase in joint temperature will not be appreciated by the examiner's hand. However, the sternoclavicular joint is superficial and an increase in temperature should be readily apparent. The patient may be examined from the front or the back, and both bony and soft tissue landmarks should be assessed.

Bony Landmarks (Figure 28A, B, C):

- sternoclavicular joint
- clavicle
- acromioclavicular joint
- coracoid process
- acromion
- spine of the scapula
- inferior edge of the scapula
- greater tuberosity of the humerus
- lesser tuberosity of the humerus

Soft Tissue Landmarks (Figure 29A, B, C):

Prominent Muscles: sternocleidomastoid, pectoralis, deltoid, biceps, trapezii, and serratus anterior
Tendons: the rotator cuff and biceps
Bursae: subdeltoid and subacromial
Also: the axilla

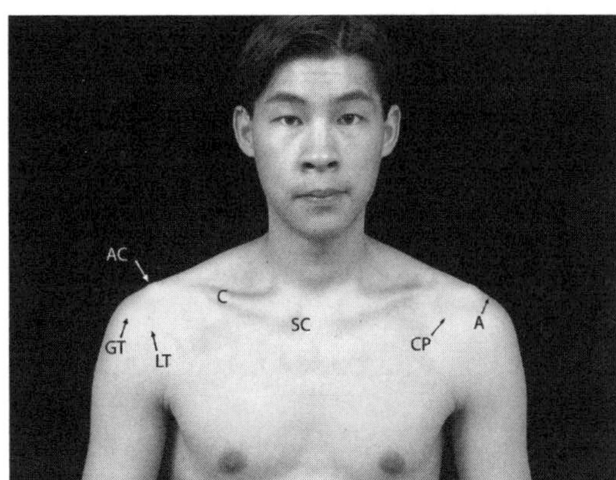

Figure 28A. A - acromion; AC - acromioclavicular joint; C - clavicle; CP - coracoid process; GT - greater tuberosity; LT - lesser tuberosity; SC - sternoclavicular joint.

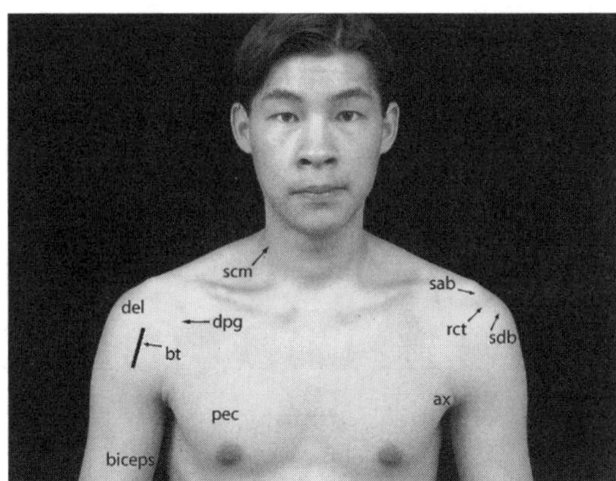

Figure 29A. ax - axilla; bt - biceps tendon; del - deltoid; dpg - delto-pectoral groove; pec - pectoralis major; rct - rotator cuff tendon; sab - sub-acromial bursa; scm - sternocleido-mastoid; sdb - sub-deltoid bursa.

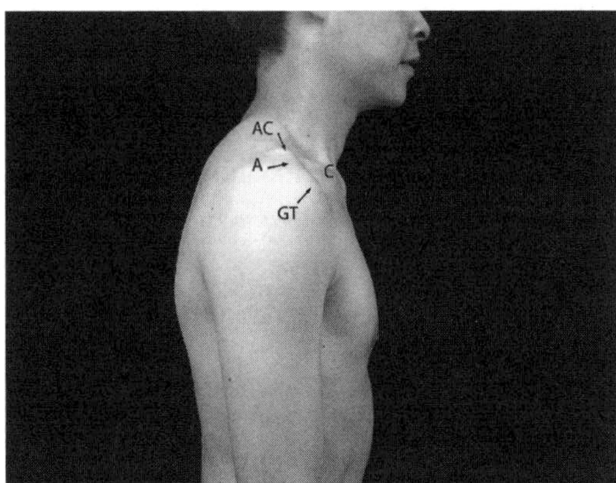

Figure 28B. A - acromion; AC - acromioclavicular joint; C - clavicle; GT - greater tuberosity.

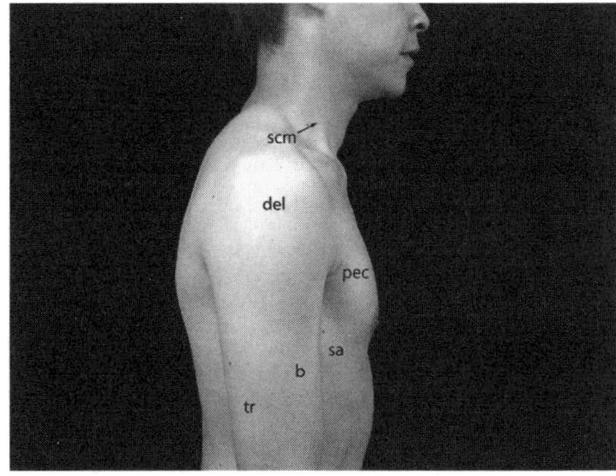

Figure 29B. b - biceps; del - deltoid; pec - pectoralis major; sa - serratus anterior; scm - sternocleidomastoid; tr - triceps.

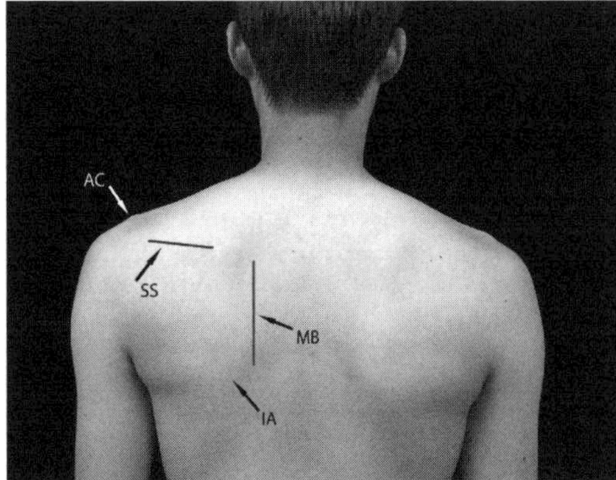

Figure 28C. AC - acromioclavicular joint; IA - inferior angle of scapula; MB - medial border of scapula; SS - spine of the scapula.

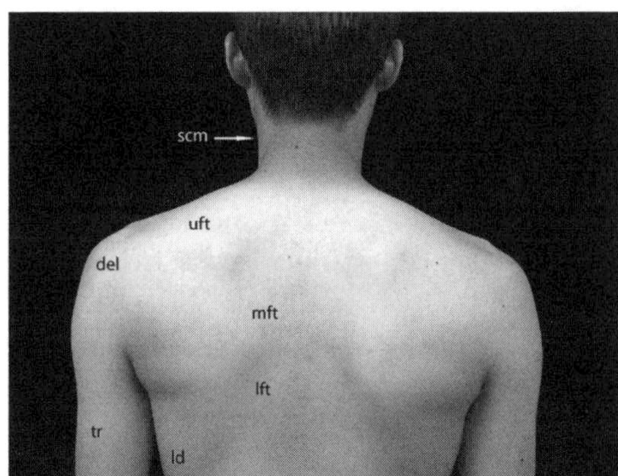

Figure 29C. scm - sternocleidomastoid; uft - upper fibers, trapezius; del - detoid; mft - middle fibers, trapezius; lft - lower fibers, trapezius; ld - latissimus dorsi; tr - triceps.

Clinical Hint:
If you experience difficulty palpating the bony landmarks because the patient has a generous amount of subcutaneous tissue (fat or muscle), identify the spine of the scapula and walk your fingers along it toward the lateral aspect of the shoulder. When you feel the bone turn the corner you have identified the posterior edge of the acromion. Keep walking your fingers toward the front of the shoulder until it turns another corner. This is the anterior edge of the acromion.

Pick a spot halfway between the anterior and posterior edge of the acromion and drop your fingers down approximately one thumb width. If you then ask the patient to externally rotate their arm, you will feel the greater tuberosity roll under your fingertips (figure 30). Just medial and anterior to the greater tuberosity is the bicipital groove whose anterior border is formed by the lesser tuberosity.

The coracoid process is separate from the humerus (remember that it is part of the scapula) and emerges slightly from under the distal end of the clavicle. It is easy to feel by cupping your hand over the shoulder, such that the ulnar edge of your palm is even with the most lateral aspect of the shoulder, and dropping your thumb down to use it to palpate just under the clavicle. You will have to lift your palm away from the shoulder to do so, but keep your fingers resting on the top of the shoulder, and you should be able to feel the bony process easily. Recall that even a healthy coracoid is quite tender on palpation.

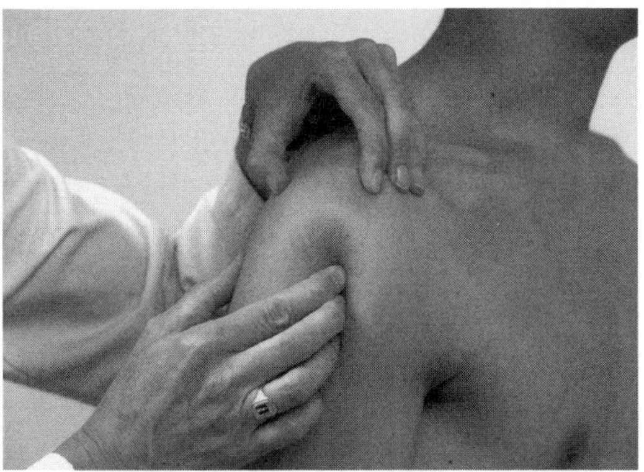

Figure 30 - Palpation of bicipital groove; the shoulder is externally rotated.

The common insertion of the posterior rotator cuff tendons can only be palpated with the shoulder in extension. Have the patient put their hand on their hip with the elbow pointing directly backwards. This brings the point of insertion out from under the roof of the acromion.

The sternoclavicular joint should be palpated for tenderness and swelling. You can accentuate the sternoclavicular joint by extending, abducting and internally and externally rotating the shoulder joint.

Range of Motion

There are six motions of the glenohumeral joint: abduction, adduction, flexion, extension, internal rotation and external rotation (figures 31A-D). The scapula, and thus the shoulder region, can also be elevated, retracted, protracted and depressed. If there is full, pain-free range of motion actively, it is unlikely that passive range of motion will yield any useful clinical information. However, if there is restriction of movement, you must check passive ROM. Make sure to look for early scapular movement; usually the scapula does not move until the humerus is abducted approximately 80-90°, and then it swings up and away. Pathology in the glenohumeral joint is frequently accompanied by early or excessive movement of the scapula.

Resisted movements are utilized to assess not only strength but also to evaluate the integrity of the tendons. If one remembers the origin and insertion of the muscles and their tendons, one can put them under a stretch or a stress; pain with either maneuver may isolate the cause of the patient's shoulder complaints. Most special tests of the shoulder exploit thisbasic principle and as such do not need to be memorized. For example, tests for bicipital tendinitis and rotator cuff tendinitis are nothing more than resisting the motion of the tendons or putting them under a stretch. If a tendon is torn, pain may not be present, but the function will be impaired; this is the principle behind the 'drop arm test'.

Special Tests

Painful Arc

Ask the patient to raise their arm over their head by lifting it away from their side (abduction) with the palm facing the ceiling during the ascent. If pain is experienced as the arm approaches the horizontal and disappears as it gets closer to the vertical, then the patient is said to have a painful arc. It implies that there is a pinching of the tissues between the humeral tuberosities and the acromion as in supraspinatus tendonitis.

Scapulothoracic and Glenohumeral Movement

Picture the shoulder joint as a 'ball and socket' joint. When the joint is healthy, there is free movement of the ball in the socket, and of the socket as part of the scapula. Normally when one lifts the arm to the side, the head of the humerus (the ball) will roll on the glenoid (the socket) and the movement will be

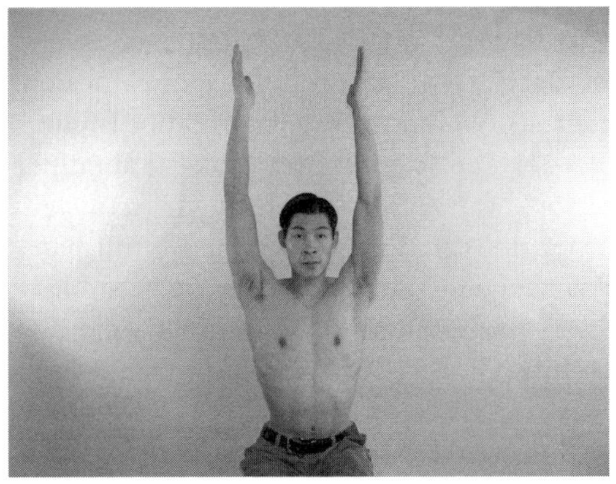

Figure 31A. Full shoulder elevation via either flexion or abduction.

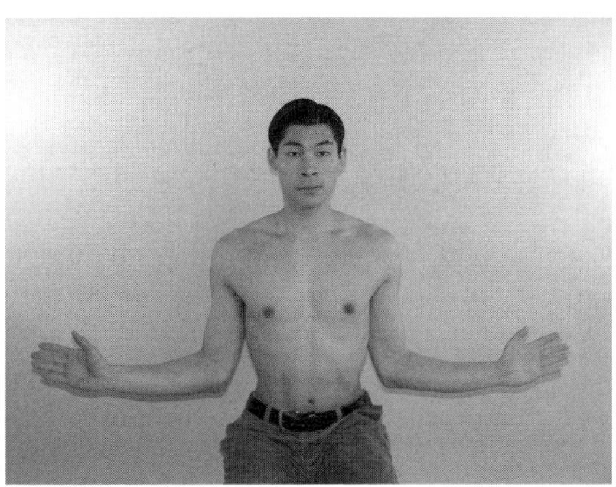

Figure 31B. Shoulder external rotation.

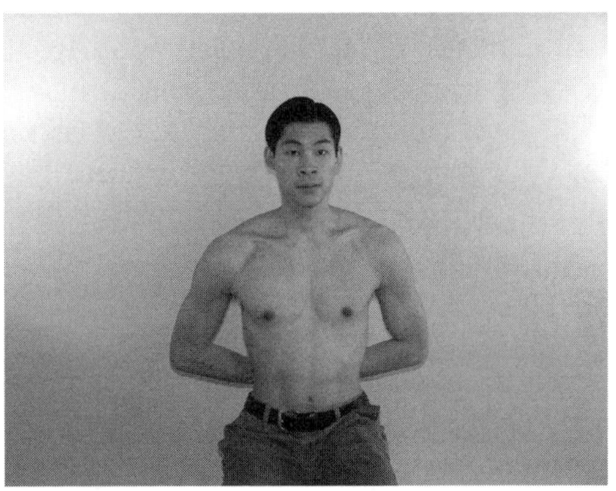

Figure 31C. Bilateral shoulder internal rotation.

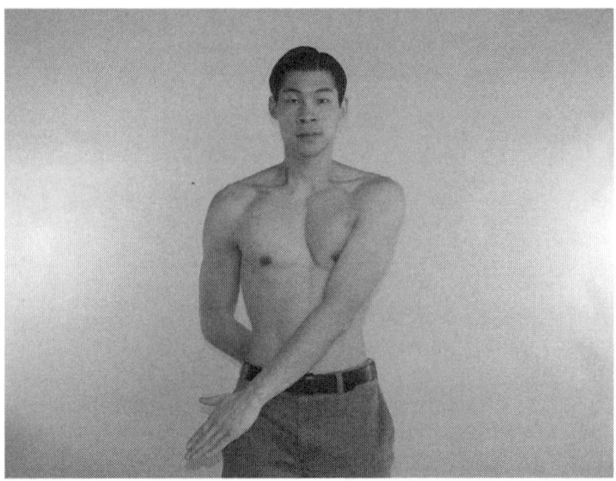

Figure 31D. Shoulder adduction.

smooth. The scapula does not move until the arm is lifted above the horizontal. If there is cause for pain in the glenohumeral joint, then the body will try to limit the movement of the humerus in the glenoid fossa of the scapula by moving the arm and scapula as a single unit. Observing the patient from the front, you will see a shrugging motion of the shoulder, but to be more precise you should palpate the inferior edge of the scapula as the patient slowly abducts the arm. Notice when you first appreciate movement of the scapula; there should be min- imal movement until the arm is raised above 75-80° at which point the scapula will 'take off'. Early scapulothoracic movement is a sign of glenohumeral joint pathology.

Drop Arm Test

This test is for tears in the rotator cuff tendons. Ask the patient to fully abduct their arm, then slowly lower their arm to their side. If the tendons are torn, the arm will drop to their side when the arm reaches approximately 90° abduction. If they can maintain their abducted arm at 90°, lightly tapping the forearm will cause the arm to drop if the tendons are ruptured.

Tests for Rotator Cuff Tendonitis/ Impingement

The rotator cuff is the primary stabilizer of the glenohumeral joint; this set of muscles also moves the shoulder through abduction and external rotation. The common tendon of the rotator cuff is vulnerable to both tendonitis and impingement along its course under the acromion. Resisted abduction with the shoulder internally rotated is used to test for pathology of the rotator cuff tendon generally, and the supraspinatus tendon specifically (figure 32). Resisted external rotation with the shoulder abducted may be used to test for impingement of the rotator cuff tendon (figure 33).

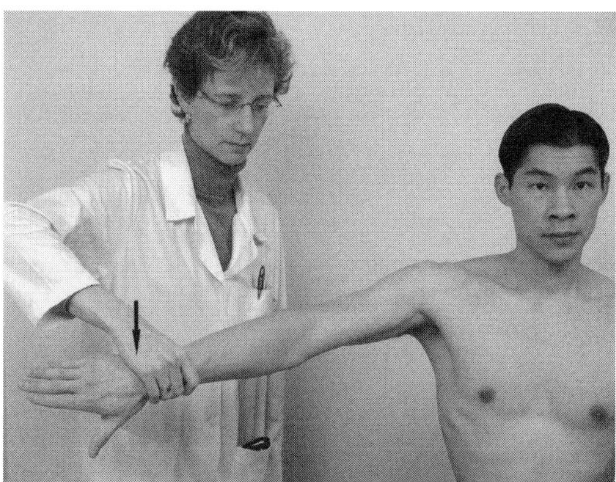

Figure 32. Resisted testing for supraspinatus tendonitis.

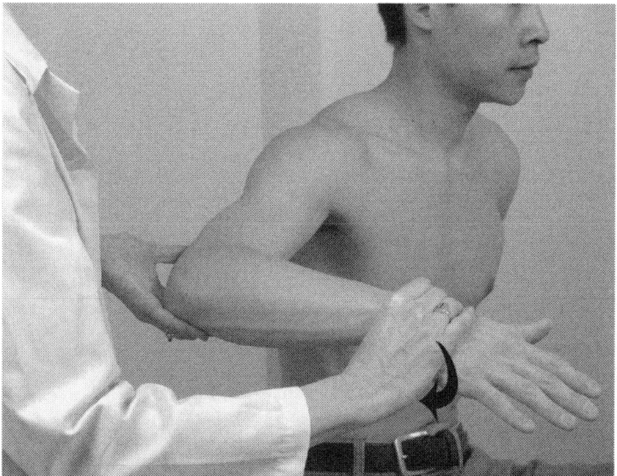

Figure 33. Resisted external rotation with the shoulder abducted tests for impingement of the rotator cuff.

Tests for Bicipital Tendonitis

Stress the bicipital tendons by resisting their primary movements: shoulder flexion, elbow flexion and forearm supination. With the shoulder in 20-30° flexion, the elbow extended and the forearm supinated, resist shoulder flexion with your resisting hand over the distal radius. The test is positive if pain is elicited in the shoulder with this maneuver (also called Speed's Test, figure 34). Stress the bicipital tendons by passively extending the shoulder and elbow, pronating and ulnar deviating the wrist (figure 35).

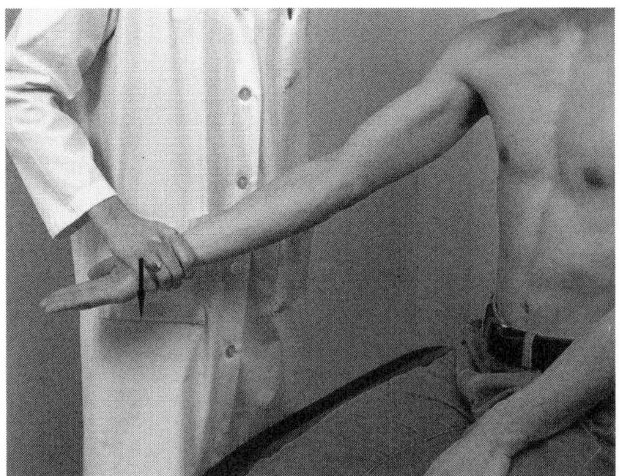

Figure 34. Resisted shoulder flexion with the elbow extended and forearm supinated tests for bicipital tendonitis (Speed's Test).

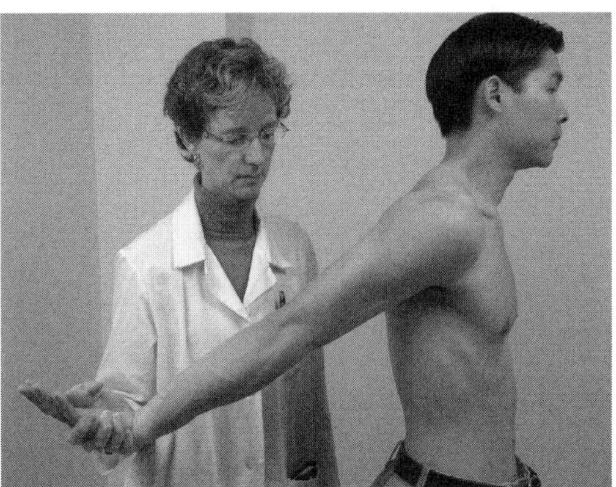

Figure 35. A passive stretch test of the bicipital tendons.

Apprehension Test for Anterior Glenohumeral Instability

Ninety five percent of dislocations of the shoulder are anterior. In patients less than 25 years of age with a first time dislocation, their risk for recurrent dislocation is as high as ninety percent. This test must be done gently and slowly. With the patient supine, support their lower arm with one hand and their upper arm with your other hand. Lift their arm away from their body (abduct) to 90°, then gradually move their arm into external rotation (figure 36).

A positive test is when the patient verbally or nonverbally expresses alarm that their shoulder feels as if it is about to dislocate. Do not persist in externally rotating the arm, as you may indeed cause the head of the humerus to dislocate.

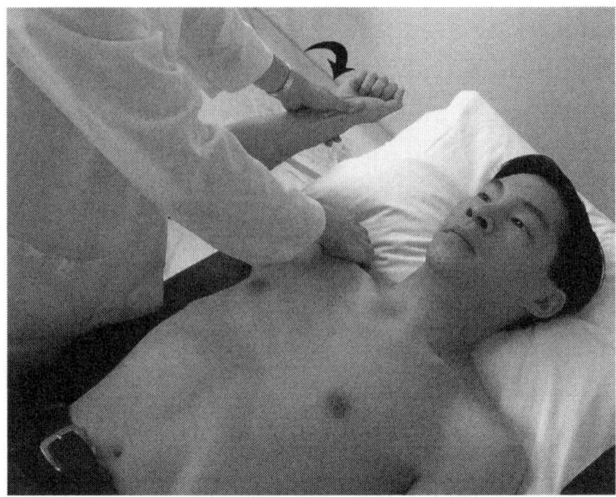

Figure 36. Apprehension Test for glenohumeral instability.

Acromioclavicular Joint Evaluation

Palpate the AC joint for tenderness and alignment. Stress the joint by compressing itwith adduction of the 90° flexed shoulder (figure 37), or with distraction forces by asking the patient to put their hand behind and across their back with the elbow extended (figure 38).

Normal exam but the patient has pain? Remember to consider referred pain from the neck or viscera. The exam is not complete until you have evaluated the cervical spine and done sensory, motor and reflex testing of the upper limb.

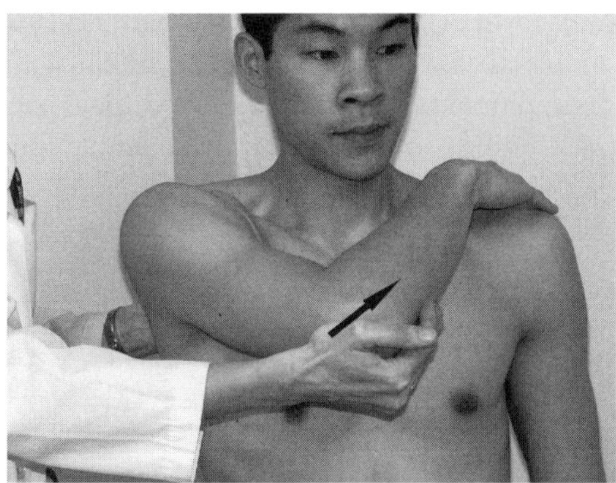

Figure 37. AC joint compression test - the shoulder is passively adducted with the shoulder at the horizontal.

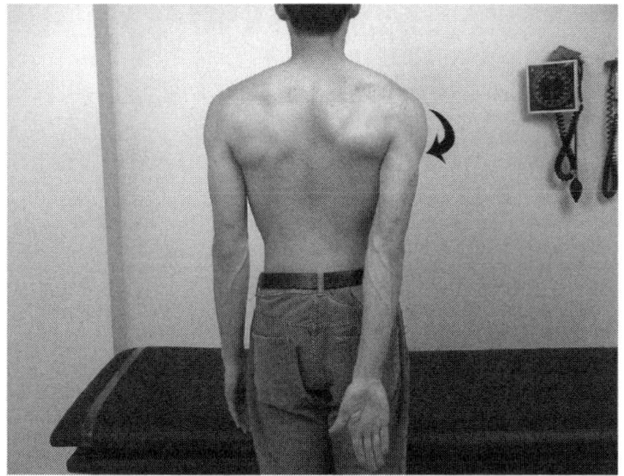

Figure 38. AC joint distraction test.

Clinical Vignettes

1. *A 52-year-old male carpet layer of 25 years, complains of right shoulder pain that is sharp and 'grabbing'. He has no pain at rest but moving his arm out to the side to put on his shirt or to reach for his tools is very painful. He cannot lie on his right arm at night to sleep. He has no other joint complaints.*

On examination of the shoulder there are no abnormalities noted on inspection. There is decreased abduction of the shoulder (actively and passively) and increased pain with resisted abduction. He has a positive painful arc test.

The diagnosis here is obvious. The patient has supraspinatous tendonitis and / or bursitis. The next question should be 'why?' Tendonitis is usually due to 'misuse, abuse or over-use' but this gentleman has been performing his occupation for many years and his muscles should be well adapted to the demands of his job. This suggests that something has changed. He needs appro- priate treatment for his shoulder, but a precipitating cause should be sought. His shoulder should be radiographed but in addition the cervical spine should be examined and x-rayed. Foraminal encroachment at C5/6 due to an osteophyte would not be unusual in this age group. This may result in weakness of the supraspinatus muscle, which sets up the tendon for increased stress. It is not enough to make a diagnosis, you should be able to explain why the problem exists.

2. *A 36-year-old male patient with HIV/AIDS complains of left shoulder pain of two weeks duration. The pain is constant and there are no alleviating features. He has had difficulty sleeping at night because of the pain. He has not had joint symptoms before, and despite his diagnosis, he has been doing reasonably well except for diarrhea that he blames on his medication. There are no associated symptoms of numbness, tingling or weakness in his left arm or other extremities.*

On examination, he is in obvious discomfort. Although he does not support his left arm with his opposite hand, he constantly moves his left arm trying to find a comfortable position. Inspection, palpation and both active and passive range of motion are normal. Resisted testing is also normal. The remainder of the MSK exam, including cervical spine and elbow examination, is normal. The neurologic examination is normal.

What is the most likely cause of this patient's pain? Trust your physical findings. You have ruled out a joint based problem for his complaints. The absence of increased pain with resisted testing points away from either a tendinous or a bone based pathology. The full range of motion tells you the glenohumeral joint is intact, without inflammation or infiltration. His normal neurologic exam goes against a neurogenic source of pain, (although not completely*) but given his history of AIDS, his risks for infection are great and you should be suspicious for referred pain from a visceral source. Since he has no respiratory complaints, and remembering that the phrenic nerve is innervated by C3, 4, and 5, look for irritiation of the diaphragm. This is an actual case of an HIV/AIDS patient with a subphrenic abscess. The key to diagnosis was found in the physical examination.

** Brachial Plexitis can be a cause of terrific shoulder pain and early on, the examination is surprisingly benign. However, with time (weeks to months) neurologic findings will develop.*

CHAPTER FIVE

Examination of the Cervical Spine

Nowhere is the dictum 'do no harm' more important than in the management of cervical spine pathology. Here, where the spinal cord is largest, the surrounding bony skeleton is stalk-like in its support of the head and has more mobility than any other region of the spine. For the purposes of this discussion, it is assumed that the examination (apart from inspection) is not in the setting of trauma, nor in a patient who describes possible vertebral-basilar insufficiency, nor in a patient with rheumatoid arthritis or some other disease process which may involve instability of the cervical spine.

Inspection

Observe the attitude of the head with respect to the torso. Is the head held in a chin forward position? If so, one might anticipate complaints of pain at the base of the neck which may radiate upwards over the occiput and be associated with tension headaches. Is the head held off to one side, or held stiffly? Make note of any scars, discoloration or swelling in the neck.

Palpation

Bony palpation should be done with the patient lying supine in order to relax the neck muscles. Identify the occiput, then palpate the spinous processes with C7 being the most prominent. Palpate the facet joints by moving your fingers about 2.5 cm (one inch) lateral to the spinous processes and press deep to the trapezius muscles. The neck muscles must be relaxed in order to appreciate the joints, which feel like small, round, hard bumps. It is not unusual to elicit tenderness but if one articulation is more tender than the others, identify the level; if you have lost count you can line up the level with the anterior structures of the neck: hyoid bone at C3, thyroid cartilage at C4 and C5, and the first cricoid ring at C6.

Range of Motion

Flexion, extension, rotation and side flexion compose the basic neck movements. Check for both quantity and quality of movement, which should be assessed actively, with reservation of passive movements for those with restricted range. Since passive range of motion requires complete relaxation of neck muscles, the patient must be supine and have complete confidence in the examiner.

Flexion: Ask the patient to look downward and touch their chin to their chest. Normal movement of the spine should allow this.

Extension: Request the seated or standing patient to bring their chin up as far as possible by tilting the head backward. The forehead should be almost parallel to the floor, and the patient should be able to look directly at the ceiling.

Rotation: Shaking your head 'no' relies on rotation of the cervical spine. Ask the patient to look to each side: the chin should be almost in line with the shoulder at end range. Make sure to assess looking both to the right and left.

Side Flexion or Lateral Bending: Ask the patient to tilt their head to bring their ear toward the shoulder. Make sure the patient does not shrug the shoulder; if necessary, place one hand on the shoulder to prevent it. Normally one should be able to tilt the head approximately 45° toward each shoulder.

Special Tests

The student is expected to be aware of the principles behind the 'compression and distraction' tests. With compression of the cervical spine, the neural foramina are narrowed, the facet joints are under increased pressure, and pain may result. If pain is localized to the neck, facet joint or disc disease may be present, but if pain is elicited in the arm or hand, foraminal encroachment of a nerve root(s) is possible. The distraction test reduces weight bearing in the cervical spine; if this maneuver reduces the patient's radiating pain, foraminal stenosis is likely.

Remember: Do not perform these tests on anyone at risk of having an unstable neck.

Compression Test

To administer the compression test, have the patient either sit or lie supine. Take care to maintain normal cervical lordosis and gently press straight down on the head. Make careful note of reports of increased pain in either the cervical spine or the arm, and determine whether it follows a dermatomal or radicular path (figure 39).

Distraction Test

The distraction test requires the patient's head to be grasped and gently drawn away from the torso. Using both hands, cup the occiput and gradually lift the head away from the torso, making sure you do not induce either rotation or side flexion as you do so. This maneuver is most easily accomplished with the patient supine. The test is considered positive for nerve root compromise when the patient's typical pain is relieved or lessened (figure 40).

Spurling's Maneuver

Compression, extension, rotation and lateral flexion of the cervical spine will elicit pain if there is prolapse of a disc or narrowing of a foramina. Ask the seated or standing patient to tilt their head to one side (lateral flexion) then lift their chin upward, as if watching a plane fly overhead, and then apply a light downward compression on their head (figure 41). Technically, compression should be maintained for ten seconds if pain is not immediately experienced. Pain will frequently be elicited in the dermatomal distribution of the compromised nerve root. Alternatively, the pain elicited may follow the path of a specific peripheral nerve, i.e., radicular pain.

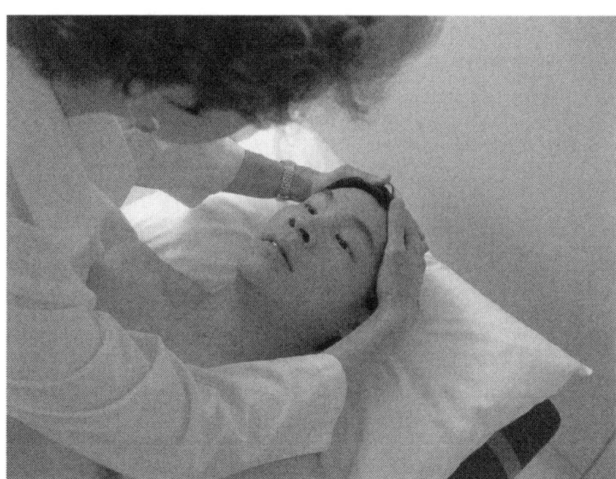

Figure 39. Cervical Compression Test.

Occiput to Wall Distance

The patient stands with their back to a wall, heels touching the base of the wall. Then ask the patient to try and touch the back of their head to the wall. A normal individual would experience no difficulties (figure 42A), but the posture of a patient with ankylosing spondylitis may become progressively more stooped, rendering this impossible (figure 42B). Serially recording the distance between the occiput and the wall with a tape measure provides useful information on the progression of the patient's disease.

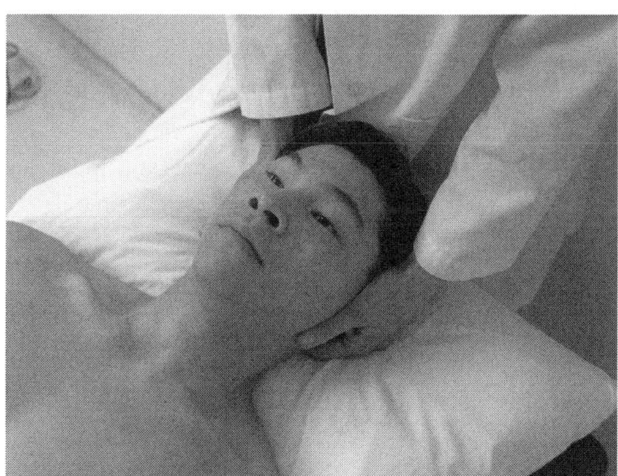

Figure 40. Cervical Distraction Test.

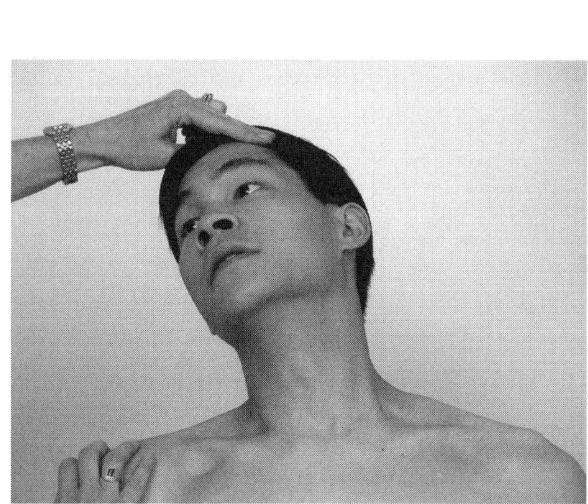

Figure 41. Spurling's Maneuver.

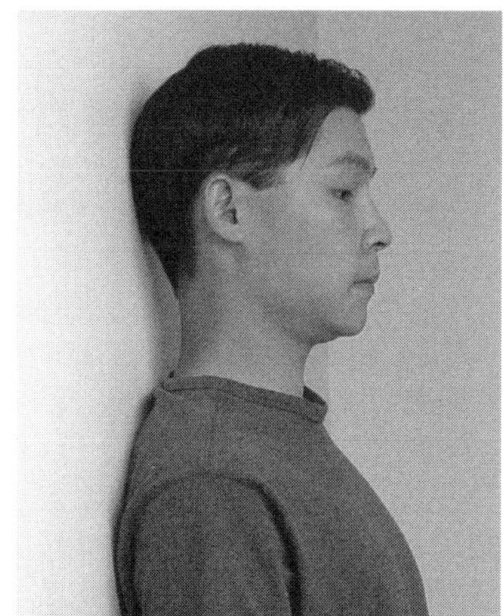

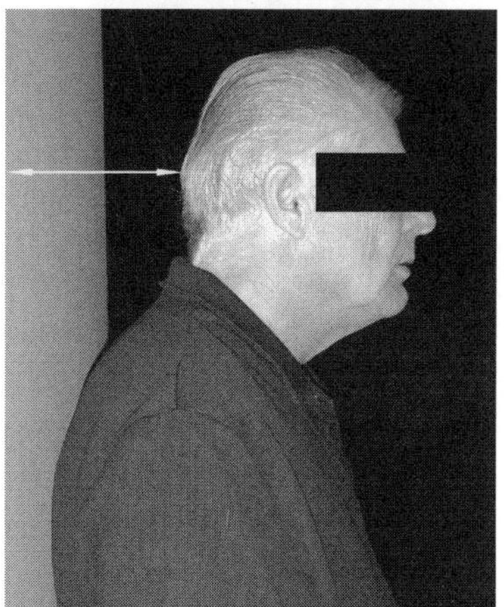

Figure 42A. (upper) Normal occiput to wall distance Figure 42B. (lower) Occiput to wall distance in the presence of ankylosing spondylitis.

Next check the deep tendon reflexes in the arms and legs and conclude with at least one test of upper motor neuron function such as the Babinski.

Clinical Vignettes

1. *A 55 year old woman with a longstanding history of rheumatoid arthritis complains of neck and occipital pain. She is particularly aware of the pain when she is trying to do needlepoint. She has not had any problems with bowel or bladder control, nor has she had any electric-like shocks down her spine or into her extremities. Her head feels "too heavy" and she finds herself unconsciously using her hand to support the weight of her head by propping up her chin.*

On examination the patient moves her head stiffly, and range is reduced in all directions. On cervical spine flexion you note that she brings her hand to her chin to support the weight of her head.

What other information would you like to obtain at the bedside, and what physical exam tests should be avoided?

The probability of instability of the cervical spine from rheumatoid arthritis is very high, and the examiner must not do any provocative compression or distraction tests, nor should the examiner perform passive movements of the neck. A neurologic exam is indicated, looking for loss of power in the extremities (frequently difficult to interpret because of rheumatoid deformities and joint pain) and absence or increase of deep tendon reflexes. The Babinski test (upgoing toes with stroking the sole or side of the foot) should also be performed. Radiographs of the cervical spine with flexion and extension views are indicated with particular attention to the C1-C2 articulation of the odontoid peg with the arch of the atlas. With flexion, normal separation of these two structures is less than 2 mm.

2. *A 36-year-old lawyer and mother of two young children complains of neck pain and burning discomfort between her shoulder blades. Symptoms have been present intermittently for years, but they have been more frequent of late. She will sometimes awaken with a very stiff, sore neck, and on those days the pain will intensify as the day progresses. Heat and massage help alle- viate the discomfort, but she is very worried about the potential significance of the burning discomfort between her shoulder blades.*

On examination the patient is tall and slim, and sits with her head in a chin-forward position. There is slight restriction of cervical spine rotation to the left and right, and on forward flexion she complains of discomfort at the base of her neck. Palpation of the para-cervical muscles and tissues (done, of course, with the patient supine) elicits pain and you note increased tone of the muscles. Neurologic examination and the remainder of the MSK exam (including lumbar examination) are normal.

In this scenario, are investigations needed? What advice would you give the patient?

This woman has mechanical neck pain, if not caused by, then certainly aggravated by poor posture. She may have early degenerative disc disease in her cervical spine, but since neither her management nor prognosis would be altered, further investigations are not recommended. Your detailed examination has ruled out sinister pathology and the patient should be reassured. It is not uncommon for burning dysesthesias to be present in a patient with mechanical neck pain and para-cervical muscle spasm. She will need assistance to correct probable life long habits of poor posture, education regarding ergonomics (e.g., carrying too much in her purse or briefcase) and would possibly benefit from stress management. Allied health professionals should be consulted for ongoing management.

CHAPTER SIX

Examination of the Lumbar Spine and Sacroiliac Joints

Not all back pain is due to pathology in the lumbar spine, and not all lumbar spine pathology will present as back pain. The history of the patient's symptoms is extremely helpful in formulating a diagnosis. Based on the patient's history, back pain can be divided into one of four types:

Mechanical: Cardinal features are symptoms worse with activity, better with rest. Stiffness is present for minutes, not hours, following prolonged inactivity.

Inflammatory: Symptoms are worse with rest, and better with activity. Stiffness is present for hours, not minutes. This is the typical pattern of the seronegative spondyloarthropathies such as Ankylosing Spondylitis.

Discogenic: Back pain may be present but generally, pain is worse in the leg in the distribution of the compromised nerve. Pain is worse with sitting, better with standing or lying down.

Pathologic: Pain is present constantly with no alleviation of symptoms with rest or exercise. Constitutional symptoms of fever or weight loss, may be present. Malignancy, infection, and referred pain from visceral sources (e.g. penetrating duodenal ulcer, aortic dissection etc.) are potential causes of this type of history, and urgent evaluation is required!

As in all aspects of medicine, the physical examination is tailored by the differential diagnosis, which is generated by a thorough history.

Inspection

Observations made as the patient walks or transitions from sitting to standing, or from lying to sitting, may provide important clues to the etiology of the patient's complaints. Anyone who has experienced significant pain in their back knows that rapid changes in position are not feasible. Is the patient walking stooped or flexed at the waist, or is there an alignment problem of the torso with the legs (a trunk shift)? Is there scoliosis of the lumbar spine, or is there a leg length discrepancy? Make note of patches of hair in the midline of the back, café-au-lait spots or other abnormalities of the skin. Normally there is mild lumbar lordosis, which may be lost in someone with mechanical or inflammatory back pain.

Palpation

To identify the bony landmarks, sit or stand behind the patient and place your fingers on the tops of the iliac crests and your thumbs on the midline of the back at the L4/L5 junction, which is at the same level as the tops of the iliac crests. The spinous processes do not over-lap at this level and mark the actual levels of the corresponding vertebral bodies, thus serving as an excellent reference point. Next, palpate the spinous processes above and below this level, looking for tenderness or obvious defects. To identify the level of the S2 spinous process, draw an imaginary line between the posterior superior iliac spines which can be located by identifying the dimples of Venus (figure 43). This line also identifies the mid portion of the sacroiliac joints.

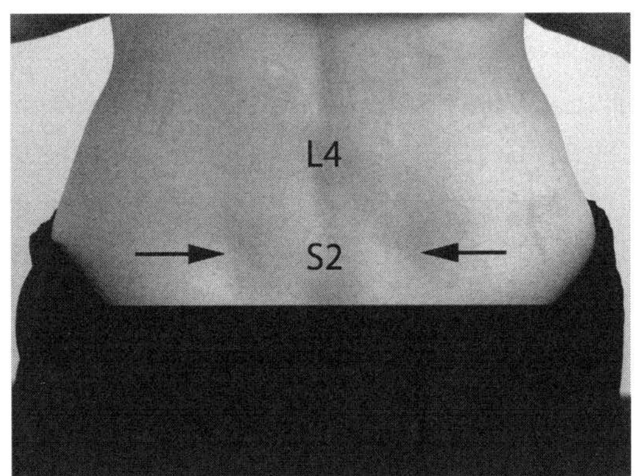

Figure 43. The location of the posterior superior iliac spines relative to S2 and L4 vertebral levels.

As a general rule, bony tenderness is specific for local pathology. Soft tissue tenderness is less specific and may be present as a component of referred pain. There is no value to palpating the paraspinal muscles when the patient is standing as they should be in a relaxed position; ask the patient to lie prone and palpate the paravertebral muscles for tenderness. Next, apply firm pressure over each sacroiliac joint to assess for tenderness (figure 44).

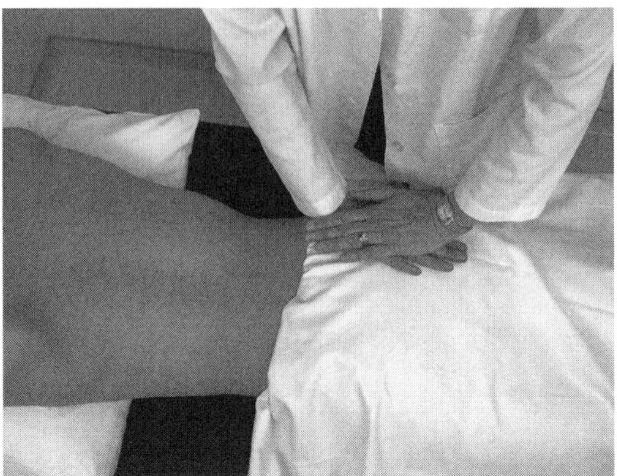

Figure 44. Assessing for tenderness at the SI Joint.

Range of Motion

The body's weight and size make passive range of motion testing in the lumbar spine arduous, so for our purposes all movement testing will be performed actively. First, have the patient extend backwards as far as possible, looking for any restriction. After returning to the upright position, check side flexion. Healthy individuals can usually touch the lateral aspect of the ipsilateral knee with full lumbar side flexion, sometimes referred to as the finger-fibula distance (figure 45).

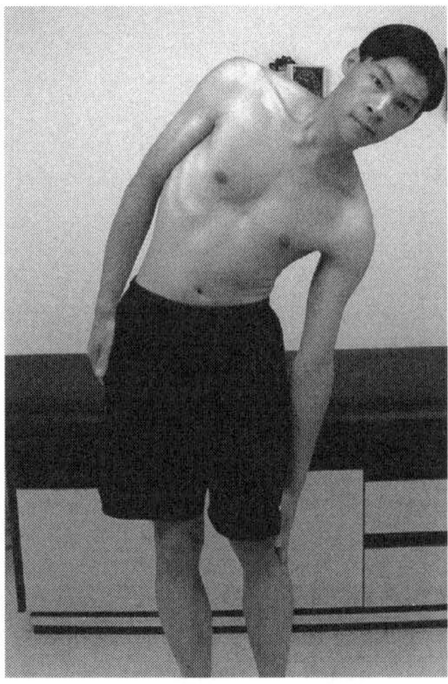

Figure 45. Assessment of side flexion using 'finger- fibula' distance.

Forward flexion is the movement most likely to be limited by a lumbar disc lesion. Some patients may not be able to flex forward at all because of intensification of the pain, others may be able to flex only with some deviation of the spine (trunk shift) which helps to reduce traction on the dura or nerve root. Early in the course of ankylosing spondylitis, restricted flexion may occur prior to radiographic changes in the lumbar spine. This is due to the inflammatory infiltrate causing stiffening of the anterior longitudinal ligament.

Rotation of the lumbar spine is negligible. The majority of trunk rotation occurs in the hips and thoracic spine. In assessing the thoracic contribution to trunk rotation, the pelvis must be stabilized; the easiest way is to have the patient sit, thus fixing the pelvis, then ask the patient to twist as far as possible to the left and then to the right.

Special Tests

Straight Leg Raising

This test evaluates the ability of the sciatic nerve, its contributing nerve roots, their dural elements and the distal extension of the sciatic nerve, the tibial nerve, to tolerate mechanical tension. It is often used to evaluate for disc herniation and nerve root entrapment. A positive SLR test along with appropriate findings on the neurological screening examination are indicative of possible nerve root compromise secondary to disc herniation.

With the patient supine, the examiner lifts the leg while maintaining knee extension. This has the effect of tensioning the various neural structures listed above, as well as the hamstring muscle. If the patient reports an increase in their symptoms, take note of the angle between the leg and the examining table; normal straight leg raising is approximately 80 - 90°. If the sciatic nerve or any of its contributing structures is compromised (often by disc herniation) pain in the lower extremity and / or back will be intensified, typically between 30 and 80 degrees of straight leg raising. If pain develops within this range, lower the leg slightly until the pain eases; this has the effect of slightly shortening the hamstrings. From this position, the foot is then dorsiflexed which further tensions the neural tissues without further stretching the hamstring muscle (figure 46). If pain is secondary to neural tissue compromise, the pain will recur with this addi- tional tensioning of the neural elements. An alternative but equivalent maneuver is to ask the patient to lift their head off the bed and tuck their chin to their chest.

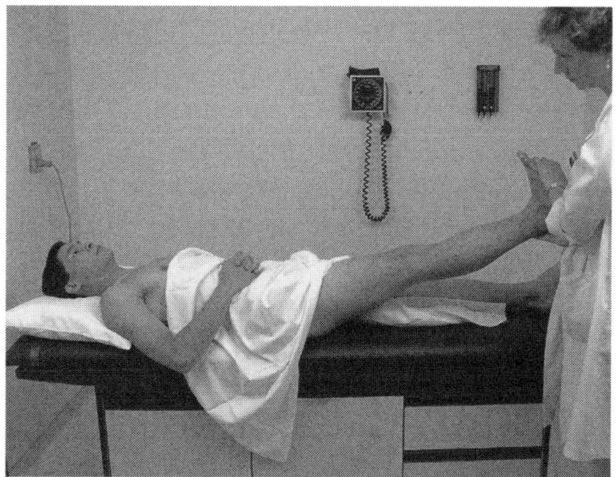

Figure 46. The Straight Leg Raise Test.

A quick test for straight leg raising (and one which may sort out those patients who may be malingering) is the Seated SLR (figure 47 - next page). With the patient seated, have them extend their knee fully or until their symptoms develop. This puts the hip and knee at 90° and the disc under compression, which will often exacerbate their pain. As with the traditional SLR, slacken the neural structures by slightly flexing the knee until the symptoms subside, then dorsiflex the ankle. If the symptoms reappear they are likely of neurogenic origin. If the patient demonstrates a normal seated SLR test but moans and groans during testing while supine, beware the malingerer.

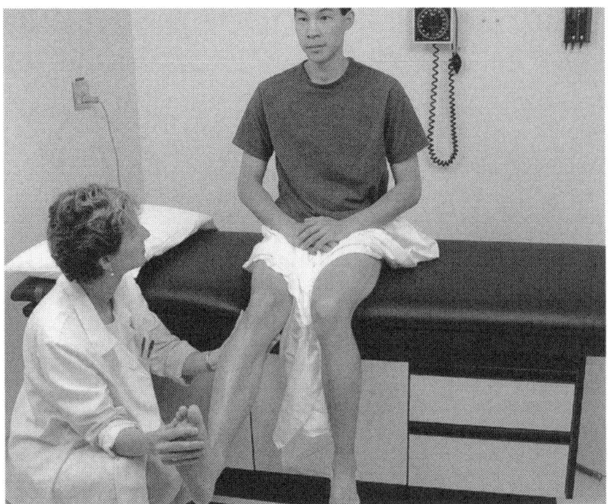

Figure 47. The Seated SLR Test.

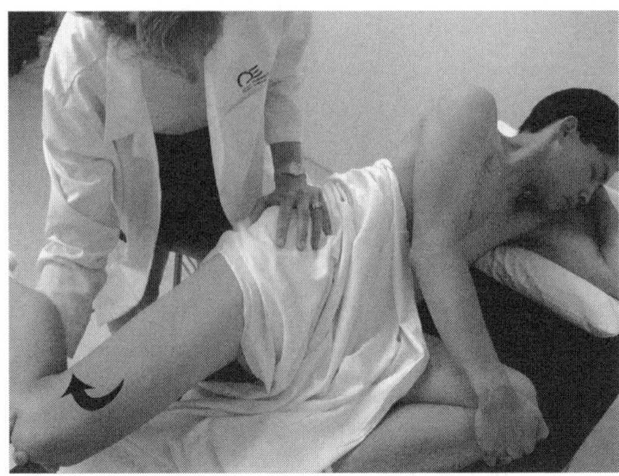

Figure 48B. Gaenslen's Test, sidelying.

Gaenslen's Test

Buttock or posterior thigh pain may originate from pathology in the sacroiliac joint. Gaenslen's test relies on the principle of pain amplification with joint stressing. The patient lies near the edge of the examination table and drops one leg over the side while flexing the other hip and knee against the chest (figure 48A). If pain is increased or elicited in the buttock of the leg hanging over the edge of the table, the test is positive and suggests sacroiliac joint dysfunction or pathology. This test can also be done with the patient lying on their side. The patient flexes their dependent leg against their chest while the clinician stabilizes the pelvis with one hand. The other hand supports the patient's lower extremity and brings the hip into extension (figure 48B).

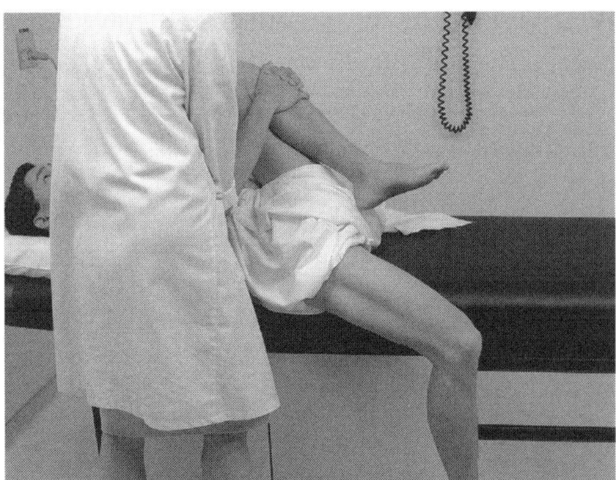

Figure 48A. Gaenslen's Test, supine.

Distraction and Compression Tests of SI Joints

These are insensitive and non-specific tests, but are used to evaluate whether SI joint pathology may be present. With the patient supine, cross your forearms, grasp the patient's anterior superior iliac spines and pull the spines toward each other. This causes a distracting force in the SI joints. Alternatively, push the anterior superior iliac spines apart, causing a compressive force within the SI joints (figure 49). Make note if the maneuvers elicit or exaggerate pain in the buttocks.

FABER Test

This is described in chapter seven (the hip) as it is more routinely used in the hip examination. However, it also creates an in- direct stress through the SI joints and is included in the evaluation of the SI joint (see page 39).

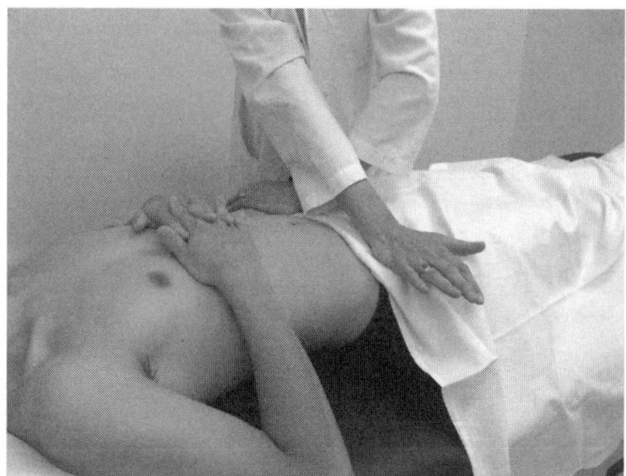

Figure 49. SI Joint Compression Test.

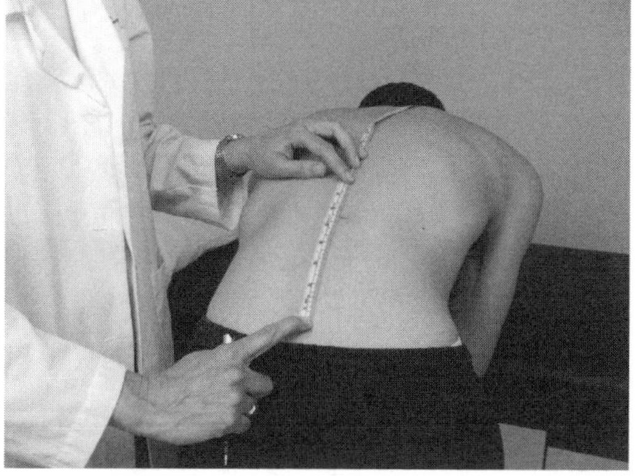

Figure 50. Modified Schober's Test.

Schober's Test

Imagine trying to bend at the waist while clasping a broomstick held vertically against your abdomen. Early in the course of ankylosing spondylitis, the anterior longitudinal ligament can become very stiff and act like that broomstick. Later in the course of the disease, there is ankylosis of adjacent vertebral bodies, which severely limits spinal mobility. Schober's test is designed to evaluate the degree of movement in the lumbar spine with forward flexion. It is done by standing behind the upright patient with their back exposed. The dimples of Venus are identified (the level of the PSIS) and a small pen mark is made on the skin 10 cm above this level. The patient is then asked to flex forward as if to touch their toes while keeping their knees straight. The distance from the line of the PSIS to the pen mark will normally increase by 5 cm. An increase of less than 4 cm suggests decreased lumbar spinal mobility (Figure 50).

If one suspects one of the seronegative spondyloarthropathies, chest expansion and occiput to wall distance should be measured.

Chest Expansion

A normal chest will move at least 5 cm from end expiration to maximum inspiration as measured with a tape measure around the chest at the level of the nipples. A measurement of 2 cm or less is said to be pathognomonic for spondylitis.

Occiput to Wall Distance

Occiput to wall distance was described as a cervical test in chapter five (page 28). However, it is also a useful test in a variety of thoracic and lumbopelvic conditions including osteoporosis-related postural dysfunctions and ankylosing spondylitis (figure 51).

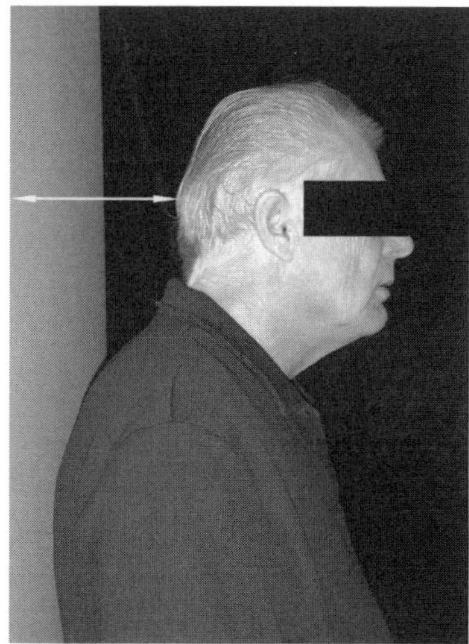

Figure 51. Occiput to wall test in a patient with ankylosing spondylitis.

Clinical Vignettes

1. *A 24 year old male sous-chef at a local hotel restaurant complains of low back pain. His job is physically demanding, requiring him to lift 100 lb bags of potatoes and large cauldrons of soups and stews, in addition to less demanding tasks. Despite this he experiences no pain at, or immediately after, work. For the past three months he has been awakening nightly with low back pain. It is so severe that he cannot get back to sleep without first getting up and walking around for approximately half an hour. When he awakens again in the morning, his back is painful again and very stiff. After two or three hours he is pain free, and he experiences no problems again until the next night.*

This young man has a classic history of inflammatory back pain. The clinician should inquire about a history of psoriasis, inflammatory bowel disease, iritis and sexually transmitted infection, in addition to a family history of inflammatory arthritis. His lumbar examination should include tests for SI joint pathology (direct and indirect stressing of the SI joints) and evaluation of the lumbar spine for loss of movement, particularly on forward and side flexion. A Modified Schober's test is essential in this scenario. At this early stage, occiput to wall distance is likely still normal, but for baseline purposes it should be recorded. You should not forget to evaluate the thoracic spine. Normal chest expansion (from end expi- ratory volume to maximum inspiratory volume) is a minimum of 5 cm. Expansion of less than 2 cm is said to be pathognomonic for ankylosing spondylitis.

2. *An 84 year old woman is brought in by ambulance from her home. She is experiencing such severe pain that she cannot move without experiencing sharp low back /posterior pelvic pain that takes her breath away. Onset was sudden and was without trauma. She had sat down rather abruptly on a kitchen chair just prior to the development of the pain, but she had not had any falls. Until now she has not had any major illnesses, and she lives alone in her own home and has been independent for self care and light housework.*

On examination, she is very alert but in terrific pain. She is lying perfectly still and says that if she moves the pain is intolerable. Her vitals are stable and she is afebrile. She can move all four limbs, but it is painful for her to move her hips. She can wiggle her toes and flex and extend her ankles without exacerbating the pain. She cannot stand or sit because of the pain.

What should your examination of the lumbar spine include?

This woman is in extreme discomfort and your examination must respect this. The most likely diagnosis is a fragility fracture of the sacrum, an unfortunate complication of severe osteo- porosis. The pain that will be present with any movement of the pelvis will limit your exam. The location of pain does not suggest hip joint pathology, but you will want to examine the lower limbs for evidence of external rotation and shortening of the limbs. Gentle palpation of the iliac crests with even gentler distraction and compression through the anterior superior iliac spines is indicated. Plane x-rays should be requested, but since sacral fractures are difficult to visualize on plane films, other diagnostic imaging will be required. On bone scan, a typical fragility fracture will light up in the shape of an 'H'. It is sometimes referred to as the 'Honda sign' because of the similarity to the shape of that company's logo. Bed rest, narcotics and intranasal calcitonin will help ease the acute pain. Long term management will require measures to address her severe osteoporosis.

CHAPTER SEVEN

Examination of the Hip

All regional exams begin with a history, and the examination of the hip is no exception. The first step is to determine whether the patient's complaints of hip pain are truly derived from the hip joint proper. Many patients are adamant that the pain is 'right in the joint' yet they will point to the lateral aspect of the hip region and/or buttock, in which case you should suspect trouble in the lumbar spine, sacroiliac joint or greater trochanter. Pain from the true hip joint (femoral-acetabular) more typically causes groin and anterior thigh pain with radiation toward the knee. Common sense should always prevail; sudden onset of severe exquisite pain, leaving an elderly patient unable to weight bear, should raise suspicion of a fracture even in the absence of trauma. Your exam in this setting should be limited to inspection and observing active range of motion until you have had opportunity to review radiographs. It is assumed for the purposes of the following discussion that fracture has been ruled out.

Inspection

Trunk shift toward the sore hip, decreased stance phase on the affected leg, and short stride length are clues to hip joint pathology. These can all be assessed by observing the patient's gait as they enter the examining room. Identify the dimples of Venus and the anterior superior iliac spines and assess whether they are in the same horizontal plane; if not, leg length discrepancy may be present. Observe the patient from the side for presence, absence or exaggeration of normal lumbar lordosis (anterior curvature of the spine). Make note of any bruises, scars, or abnormal swelling.

Palpation

Identify the following bony landmarks:

- anterior superior iliac spines
- iliac crest
- greater trochanter
- ischial tuberosity

Both the ischial tuberosity and the greater trochanter are easier to palpate with the hip flexed. Exquisite tenderness may be due to bursitis or enthesitis (inflammation of tendons where they insert into bone).

Soft tissue landmarks:

- femoral artery
- inguinal ligament
- trochanteric bursa

Make note of enlarged lymph nodes and of soft tissue swelling. Recall that not all groin pain is hip pain.

Range of Motion

Observation of active range of motion is not particularly accurate in the hip. For example, if you evaluate motion with the patient standing, the pelvis will not be fixed, making it easy to miss a flexion contracture. Conversely, problems with balance may mislead you to assume that there are problems with the hip although there are none. As a quick screen for active range of motion, observe the patient's gait, have them sit and cross their legs and then perform a full squat from standing. The full squat is a good screening test for hip joint pathology; if a patient can fully squat without shifting their weight to the non-painful side, they are unlikely to have any true hip joint pathology. Once these screening tests are completed, move on to passive range of motion testing.

The hip is a ball-in-socket joint like the shoulder and one can correctly anticipate that there are similarities in movement. Abduction, adduction, flexion, extension, internal rotation and external rotation are the movements at the hip joint. However, unlike the shoulder, the body demands that the hip remain stable; hence the amount of movement in each direction is markedly less than at the shoulder. There are similarities between the femur and the humerus, but their articulating partners, the pelvis and scapula, differ importantly in terms of mobility. The scapula is allowed to swing away from the trunk, but catastrophic trauma would be required for the pelvis to do so. However, the hemipelvis can move up and down as a unit. Indeed, jazz and hip-hop dancers utilize exaggerated movements of the hemipelvis for some of their dance moves; strong hip abduc- tors are a necessity for them.

Hip Abduction

With the patient lying supine, grasp the patient's ankle with one hand and firmly rest your other hand on the opposite anterior superior iliac spine. Gently pull the leg away from the midline as far as it will go (figure 52). Test both legs and compare. Normal abduction is approximately 45 - 50°.

Hip Adduction

Continue to stabilize the pelvis and guide the leg across the midline of the body and over the opposite leg (figure 53). Normal adduction is 20°. Repeat the maneuver for the opposite leg and compare.

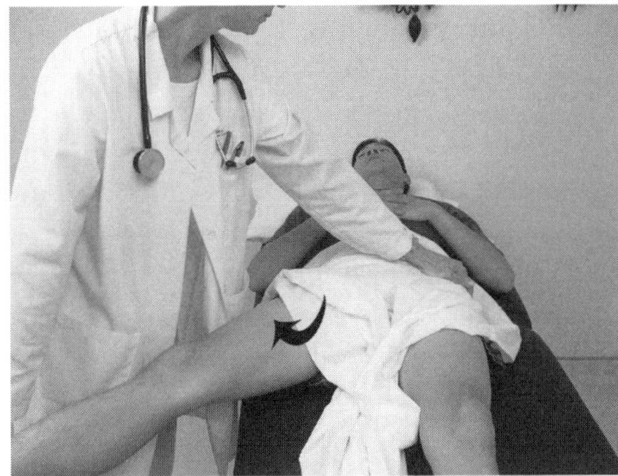

Figure 52. Passive Hip Abduction.

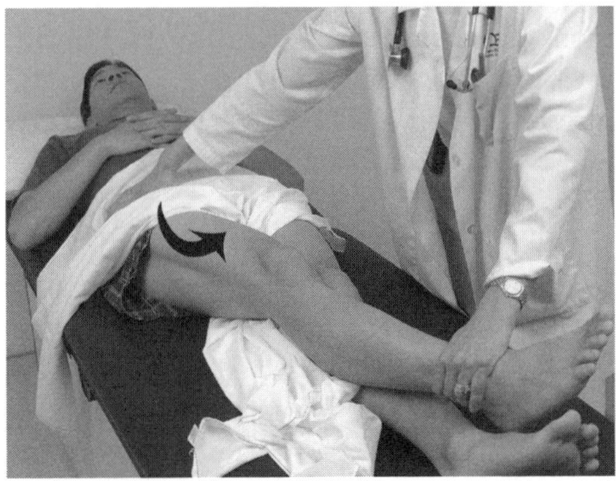

Figure 53. Passive Hip Adduction.

Hip Internal And External Rotation

One should test the range of femoral rotation with the hip in both the flexed and neutral (extended) positions. With the patient supine, stand at the side of the bed and grasp the patient's lower leg just above the malleoli. Roll the leg inwards and outwards, using the patella as a guide to evaluate range (this is sometimes referred to as 'log rolling'). One can evaluate both legs simultaneously if you wish.

Next, check internal rotation with the hip and knee flexed (figure 54). Cup the heel in your hand and use your other hand as a guide at the knee to prevent the leg from 'flopping' into abduction or adduction. Gently bring the foot laterally away from the midline to test internal rotation; bring the foot medially inwards to test external rotation (figure 55 - the apparent reversal of these movements is due to the hip being flexed during the test). Normal ranges are 35° internal rotation and 45° external rotation.

Hip Flexion

Ask the patient to flex their hip as far as it will go while he / she is lying supine; normal flexion will allow the hip to bend greater than 120° and the anterior thigh will touch the abdomen and chest (figure 56). Abdominal pannus (present in the morbidly obese patient) may obstruct hip flexion and note should be made of the actual number of degrees of hip flexion.

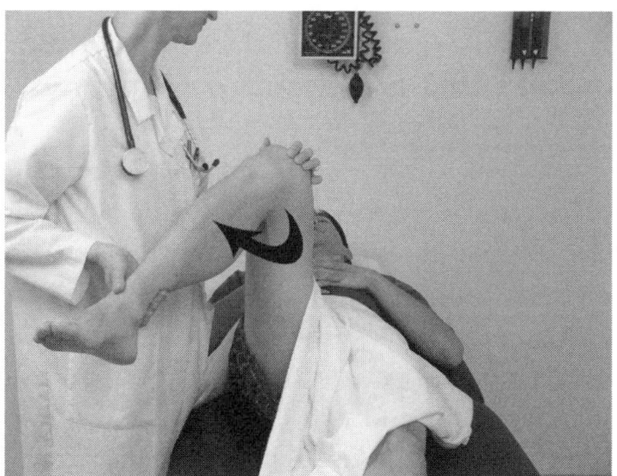

Figure 54. Passive Hip Internal Rotation.

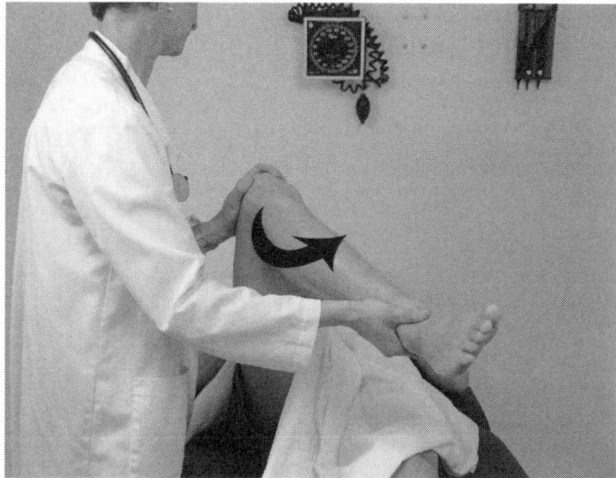

Figure 55. Passive Hip External Rotation

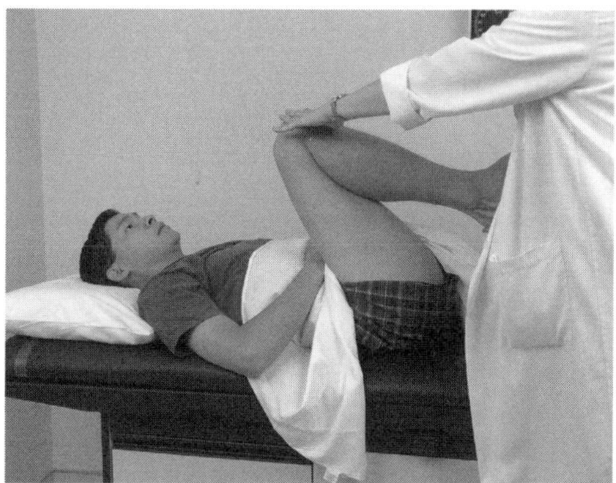

Figure 56. Passive Hip Flexion.

Hip Extension

To assess extension, the pelvis must be fixed in position. Have the patient lie prone and stabilize the pelvis with one hand over the posterior iliac crest and lumbar spine. Ask the patient to flex their knee, put your other hand under their thigh and gently lift upward (figure 57, next page). Expect 20 to 30° in a normal hip.

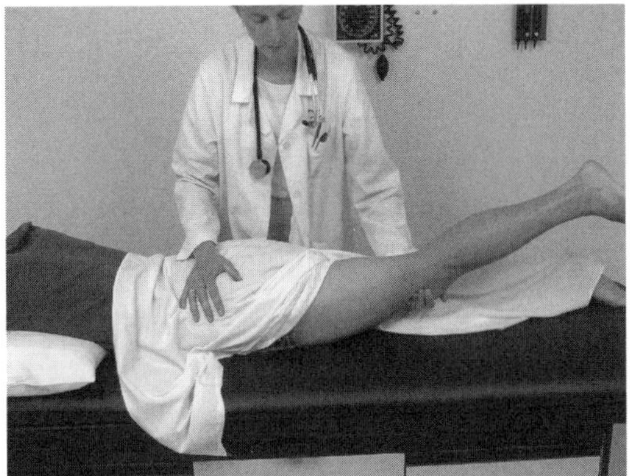
Figure 57. Passive Hip Extension.

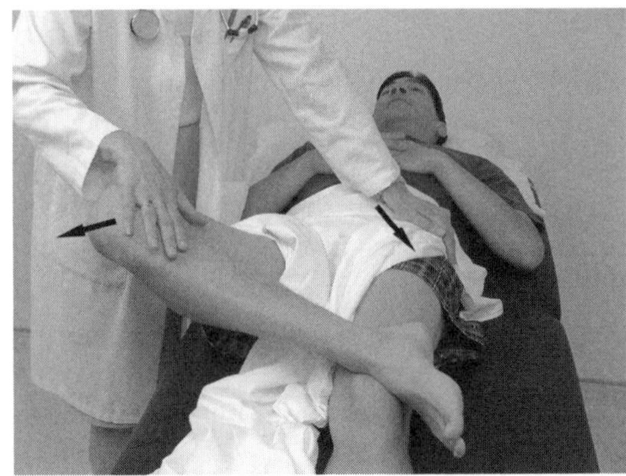
Figure 58. FABER Test.

Special Tests

FABER Test (Patrick's Test)

Information may be gleaned about the status of the hip and sacroiliac joint with this test. FABER is a pneumonic for the components of the test:

- F Flexion
- AB Abduction
- ER External Rotation

Have the patient lie supine and place the lateral malleolus of the leg being tested on the opposite knee. The hip joint will now be flexed, abducted and externally rotated. Next place one hand on the flexed knee, the other hand on the opposite anterior superior iliac spine and gently press down with both hands (figure 58). Pain in the groin suggests hip joint or surrounding muscle pathology and will usually be present without the addition of pressure at the pelvis and knee. Pain in the buttock is suggestive of problems in the sacroiliac joint.

Thomas Test

This is a simple test for hip flexion contracture. Place one hand under the patient's lumbar spine and ask the patient to draw their opposite hip to their chest (figure 59). This will eliminate the patient's lumbar lordosis; the small of their back will press into your hand. If a flexion contracture is present the contralateral leg will lift off the bed. The angle between the examining surface and the femur indicates the degree of hip flexion contracture.

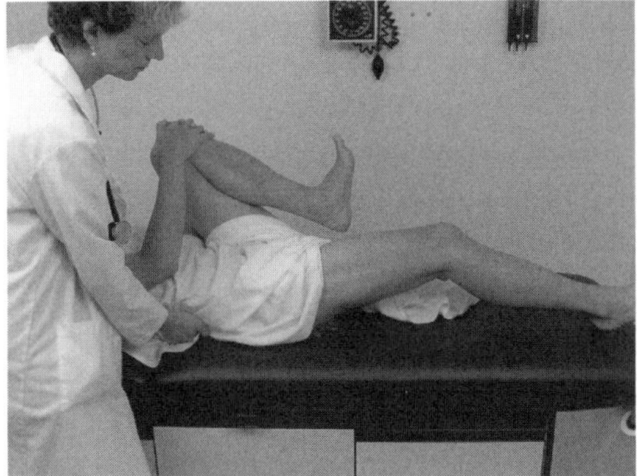
Figure 59. Thomas Test.

Trendelenburg Test

This test is designed to evaluate the strength of the hip abductors, particularly the gluteus medius muscle. Stand behind the patient and identify the 'dimples of Venus' (dimples overlying the posterior superior iliac spines). In the normal individual they appear level. Next ask the patient to lift one heel towards you such that they are standing on one leg.

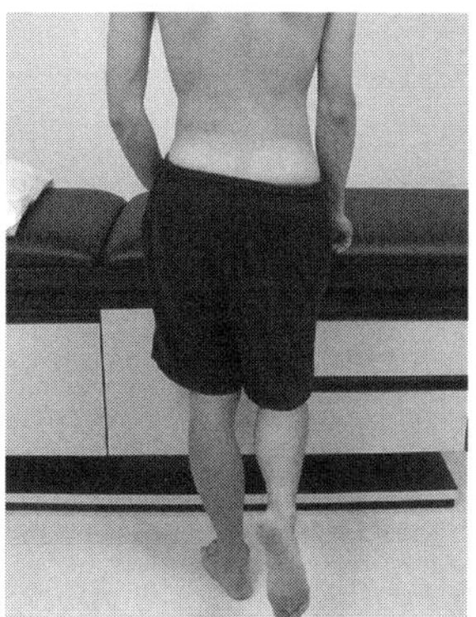

Figure 60. Trendelenburg Test.

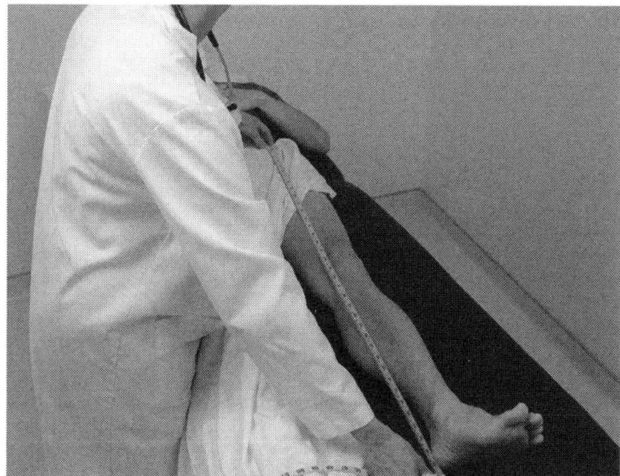

Figure 61. Leg Length Testing.

The pelvis will elevate slightly on the lifted leg side because of contraction of the gluteus medius muscle on the weight bearing side. If there is weakness of the weight bearing-side gluteus medius, the non-weight bearing side of the pelvis will drop (figure 60). There are a number of potential causes for weakness of the gluteus medius, including congenital dislocation of the hip, slipped capital femoral epiphysis, fracture of the greater trochanter, nerve root impingement, and other neuromuscular causes.

Leg Length Discrepancy

Leg length discrepancy may be true or only apparent. Apparent leg discrepancies may result from a flexion contracture of the knee or hip or may be due to pelvic obliquity. To evaluate true leg length, have the patient lie supine and measure from the notch just below the anterior superior iliac spine to the bottom of the calcaneus (figure 61). Some texts advise measuring to the medial malleolus, but if the patient has significant subtalar disease, a true leg length discrepancy will be missed; therefore, measuring to the bottom of the calcaneus is recommended. If there is a discrepancy it will be in the femoral or tibial component of the leg. With the patient supine, have them flex their knees such that their feet are flat on the table and their heels together, level at the heels. If the knee is higher on one side, that lower extremity's tibia is longer. If the femur is longer, the knee will project further anteriorly.

If there is no true leg length discrepancy but there appears to be a difference in the length of the legs, it may be due to pelvic obliquity and the anterior or posterior spines will appear uneven when the patient is standing. Measure from the xiphisternal junction or from the umbilicus to the medial malleolus of each leg and compare. Unequal distances signify apparent leg length discrepancy if true leg length measurements are equal.

Gait Assessment

A detailed discussion of gait analysis is beyond the scope of this manual; the interested reader is encouraged to review the relevant chapters in either *Physical Examination of the Spine & Extremities* by Stanley Hoppenfeld, or *Orthopaedic Physical Assessment* by David McGee. At a minimum, however, the student should be aware of the stance and swing phases of the normal walking cycle and the components of each. Clinicians should appreciate that pain, weakness and problems with balance may affect one or both phases of the gait cycle.

Stance Phase

The weight bearing portion of the walking cycle is called the stance phase, and is divided into the following components: initial contact, midstance, terminal stance and pre-swing.

When someone has a sore foot, ankle, knee or hip they will typically spend less time weight bearing through the painful extremity. In an attempt to alleviate the pain they adopt an **antalgic gait** (limp), spending as little time as possible in the stance phase of gait. By observing which component of stance phase is most dysfunctional one may be able to determine the cause of the problem. For example, a person with a sore great toe might have normal initial contact and midstance phases, but their pre-swing phase of gait is affected. The individual with a sore knee will walk with their knee semi-flexed and have little to no heel strike at initial contact. Notice the width of the patient's stance; a wider than average base of support may reflect problems with balance, coordination or lack of confidence with footing.

Swing Phase

Swing phase occurs when the foot is moving forward and is not in contact with the ground. Three components of swing phase are described: initial swing, midswing and terminal swing. Muscle weakness may affect one or all three components. Examples of weakness causing an abnormal gait are the characteristic high stepping gait of someone with 'foot drop' from a peroneal nerve palsy and the exaggerated rise and fall of the hemipelvis in a patient with a Trendelenburg gait. In summary, the analysis of gait is not just a component of the hip examination, but is an integral component of the general examination. Recognition that a patient's gait is abnormal may be the first step in determining the etiology of a patient's problem.

Clinical Vignettes

1. *A 55-year-old woman presents with complaints of left hip pain. The pain is over the lateral aspect of the hip region and it radiates laterally down the thigh to just above the knee. Onset was insidious but dates to at least two months ago. She has no problems walking, but she experiences significant discomfort in getting out of low chairs, swinging her leg to get out of her car, and climbing stairs. Pain over the side of her hip awakens her if she rolls onto her left side. She is otherwise well.*

This scenario is very typical for trochanteric bursitis. It is frequently seen in middle aged to elderly individuals, more frequently in women. It may represent a true bursitis or inflammation of the gluteus maximus and medius muscle tendons. The physical examination is usually diagnostic; there is tenderness over the greater trochanter and frequently, the surrounding muscle as well. Range of motion of the hip is not usually restricted unless the patient also has hip osteoarthritis. External rotation and resisted abduction of the hip may exacerbate the pain.

2. *You are asked to see a 45-year-old male in the coronary care unit for evaluation of severe left hip pain. He is receiving intravenous heparin in addition to multiple anti-anginal agents. Pain began in his left groin and anterior thigh approximately 24 hours ago, and the discomfort is worsening. He is aware of altered sensation over the front of his thigh - he has difficulty describing it, but it feels almost numb.*

He is not allowed to stand (in fact the pain is so great he would not wish to do so). On inspection, he is lying uncomfortably in bed, but there is no leg length discrepancy. He is able to flex, abduct and adduct his hips, but all movements of the left hip are painful. He cannot extend his hip (tested with him lying on his right side), and it is very apparent that any attempts to extend the hip actively or passively result in extreme pain. The *Thomas*

Test is suggestive of a flexion contracture of the left hip.

This gentleman should be considered to have a retroperitoneal bleed until proven otherwise - his heparin must be discontinued. He is at risk for permanent femoral nerve injury. He is holding his hip in slight flexion as this eases the pressure on the iliopsoas muscle. Extension of the hip stretches both the ilio-psoas and the femoral nerve, causing increased discomfort.

CHAPTER EIGHT

Examination of the Knee

Of all the peripheral joints, the knee may be the most common cause of complaint. Athletic injuries, simple falls, mal-alignment and/or tracking problems of the patella and osteoarthritis cause the majority of knee pathology. However, it is also a popular target in virtually all of the inflammatory arthropathies, from crystal induced to seronegative and seropositive diseases. Conversely, knee pain may be the only symptomatic expression of hip disease; in this case, the knee exam is normal while the hip exam is not.

Inspection

Observation of the patient's gait is the first step in the knee examination. A sore knee may declare itself with an antalgic (pain relieving) gait. Typically, there will be decreased stance phase on the affected side if the weight bearing portion of the knee is affected, but there may be no alteration in weight bearing time if the patellofemoral joint is the cause of discomfort. In this case, look instead for shorter stride length. Remember that hip joint pathology will typically result in a trunk shift towards the sore limb. With the patient standing, evaluate the femoral-tibial articulation. Is there an abnormal angulation of the femur with respect to the tibia? Look specifically for varus (bowleg), valgus (knock-knee) and genu recurvatum (sway-back knee) deformities. Make note of surgical scars and look for signs of muscle wasting in the quadriceps group of muscles. Isolated atrophy of the vastus medialis muscle is a consistent indication of articular knee pathology at either the femoral-tibial joint or the patellofemoral joint.

A joint effusion may be appreciated by loss of the normal indentation along the medial aspect of the knee adjacent to the patella. The suprapatellar pouch normally extends approximately ten cm above the superior pole of the patella; it may be very prominent and appear full in a moderately or grossly swollen knee.

Palpation

Temperature

Even on a warm summer day, a normal knee joint should feel cool to the examiner's touch. If the knee feels as warm or warmer than the ipsilateral thigh muscles it is a 'hot joint' and one would expect to find signs of increased joint fluid or of proliferative synovium as seen in rheumatoid arthritis. Osteoarthritic knees may have increased amounts of fluid, but typically the joint will be cool. Palpate lightly with the ulnar aspect of the palm or wrist and compare the temperature of the knee to the thigh muscles and to the opposite knee.

Fluid

Next assess for increased fluid in the joint. A small effusion may be detected by looking for the Bulge Sign (figures 62A and 62B). Picture the joint capsule as a sac-like structure; if there is a lot of fluid, the sac will be big and round, while if there is just a moderate amount of fluid, the sac will have a bulge where the fluid collects. The bulge sign relies on the clinician's ability to 'milk' the fluid from one part of the knee to the other and observe the resultant 'wave' of fluid. There is more than one way to do this test, but one of the easiest is as follows:

First, 'milk' all the fluid from the medial compartment of the knee upwards into the supra patellar pouch (figure 61A). Then milk the fluid back into the medial compartment (figure 61B). Keep your eyes trained on the medial compartment to see if you can see the fluid wave. If you can, the test is positive. If a fluid wave cannot be observed, either there is no effusion or there is such a large effusion that the sac was full and the fluid could not be moved from one compartment to the other. Usually one can easily tell the difference in the thin legged individual but the morbidly obese patient presents a challenge. A large effusion distends the joint capsule in a global fashion and one will be unable to milk fluid from one compartment to the other. Pressing down on the patella and then quickly releasing it results in the patella bouncing back into position. This test is not very helpful in the obese patient who may have a generous retro-patellar fat pad. Instead, the following is recommended: gently rest your fingers on either side of the knee below the mid portion of the patella, then with the other hand press down on the patella. If there is a large effusion you will feel the fluid push against your sensing fingers on either side of the knee joint. You can also appreciate a large effusion by pushing fluid from one side of the knee to the other. Use both hands, with fingers on one side of the knee and thumbs on the other, to push the fluid medially and laterally. A grossly swollen knee will have so much fluid that you will be unable to move fluid from one compartment to the other but you will feel the transmitted pressure; it feels like a distended, overfilled balloon.

Once you have completed assessment for warmth and fluid, identify the important soft tissue and bony landmarks of the knee (figures 63-65, next page). Palpate the knee, looking for tenderness of the soft tissue structures or bony landmarks as noted above. Tenderness

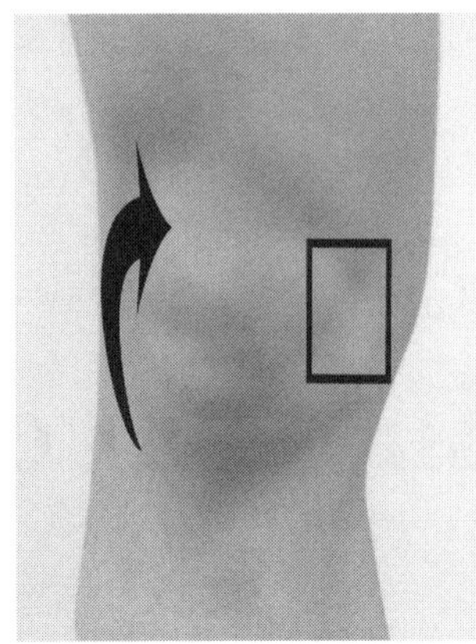

Figure 62B. Bulge Sign Phase 2: the arrow indicates the direction of 'sweep' used to bring any effusion towards the medial aspect of the knee. The clinician observes the area within the box for signs of a 'fluid wave' moving to the medial aspect.

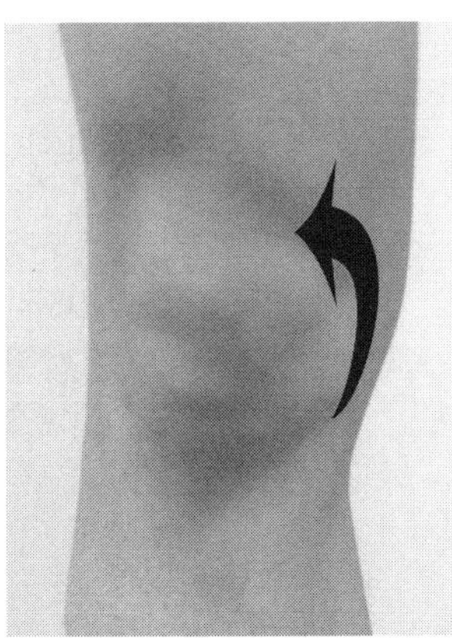

Figure 62A. Bulge Sign Phase 1: the arrow indicates the direction of 'sweep' used to bring an effusion from the medial aspect of the knee toward the suprapatellar pouch.

Soft Tissue and Bony Landmarks of the Knee

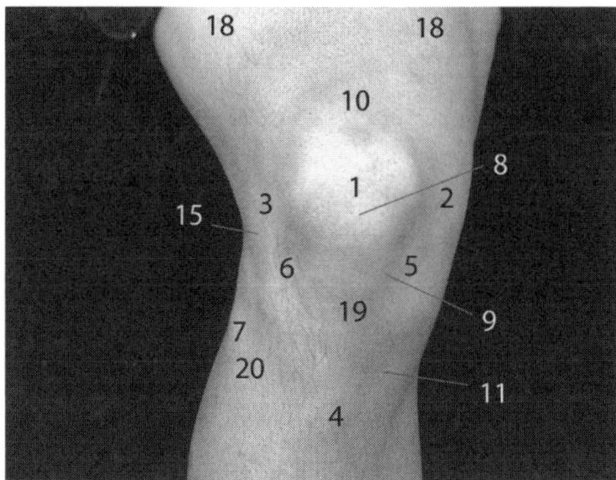

Figure 63. Right knee, anterior view.

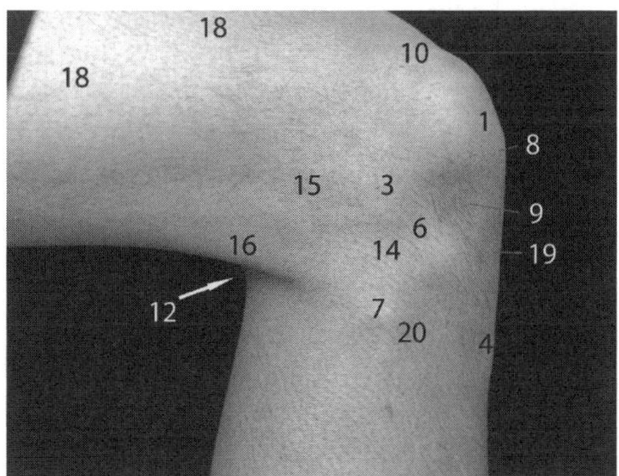

Figure 64. Right knee, lateral view.

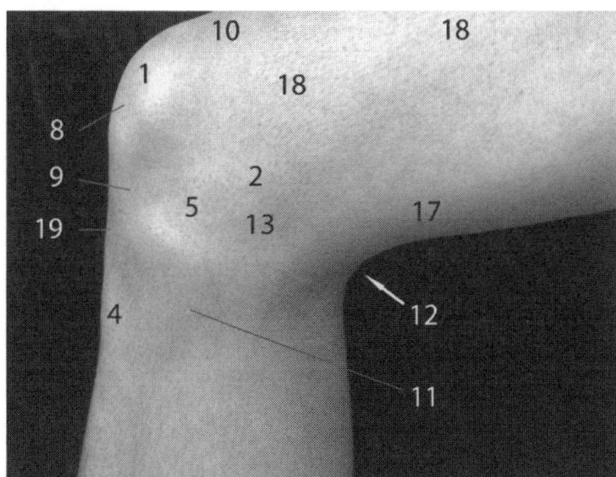

Figure 65. Right knee, medial view.

Bony Landmarks

1. patella
2. medial femoral condyle
3. lateral femoral condyle
4. tibial tuberosity
5. medial joint line
6. lateral joint line
7. fibular head

Soft Tissue Landmarks

8. prepatellar bursa
9. infrapatellar bursa
10. suprapatellar bursa
11. anserine bursa
12. popliteal fossa
13. medial collateral ligament
14. lateral collateral ligament
15. illiotibial band
16. biceps femoris
17. medial hamstrings and sartorius
18. quadriceps muscle
19. patellar tendon
20. peroneal nerve

along the medial or lateral joint line may reflect cartilaginous damage, meniscal derangement or an arthritic process. Tenderness of the bursa may reflect bursitis; a frequently overlooked cause of medial knee pain is anserine bursitis. In addition to tenderness, look for signs of swelling.

Remember that isolated soft tissue tenderness is very non-specific. In addition to bursitis, local pathology in the blood vessels, skin, nerves or fat, even referred pain from the spine, can manifest as localized tenderness. Always look for the 'best fit' of clinical and physical findings in formulating a diagnosis.

Range of Motion

The knee joint is a hinge joint and the two most important motions are flexion and extension. One would have difficulty operating foot pedals on a piano (among other things) if there was not also an element of inversion (inward rotation) and eversion (outward rotation) of the tibia with respect to the femur.

Normal range of motion of the knee is from 0° extension to 135° flexion. The tibia may also rotate relative to the femur from 10° inversion to 10° eversion.

Special Tests

Stability

The joint capsule, the anterior and posterior cruciates, and the medial and lateral collateral ligaments, in addition to the muscles that cross the knee joint, are responsible for stability of the knee. The following tests are frequently used to evaluate the integrity of the ligamentsof the knee. Bear in mind that no test is 100% sensitive. In the acutely injured knee, one is more likely to have false negatives than positives (secondary to the pseudo-stability afforded by moderate to large effusions). Likewise, the tests may be uninterpretable because pain may inhibit the patient from allowing you to do the tests adequately.

Collateral Ligaments

With the knee semi-flexed to approximately 30°, apply a varus force to the knee to test the integrity of the lateral collateral ligament and a valgus force to the knee to test the medial collateral ligament. While this sounds simple, it may be awkward, particularly if the patient is quite large.

Better control of the knee is developed if the patient is lying supine with the knee slightly flexed. Grasping the lower leg with one hand, place your other hand on the side of the knee (medial or lateral) opposite to that which you intend to test. Cup the patient's lower leg, lightly grasping the calf with one hand and your forearm supporting the weight of the leg. In this position it is easy to hold the ankle against your body with your elbow and use the patient's leg as a lever to apply force through the knee joint (figure 66).

To test the medial collateral ligament, apply a valgus force by levering the leg such that the force is outwards on the lower leg and inward at the knee joint. With the knee flexed to 30°, grasp the lower leg as described above and apply a force through your other hand just above the lateral aspect of the knee. This centers the force of the lever through

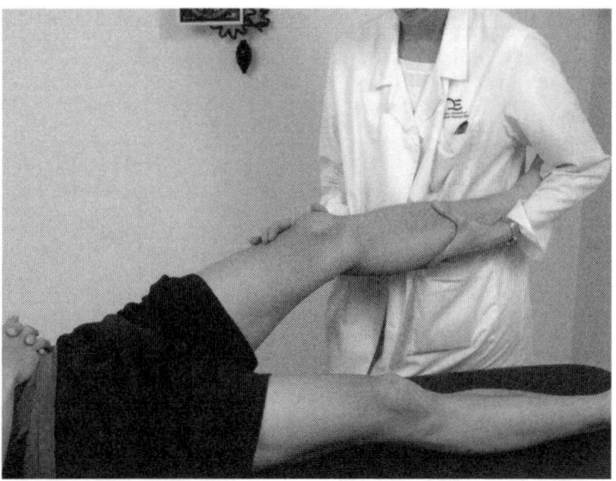

Figure 66. Correct handling in preparation for testing of the medial collateral ligament

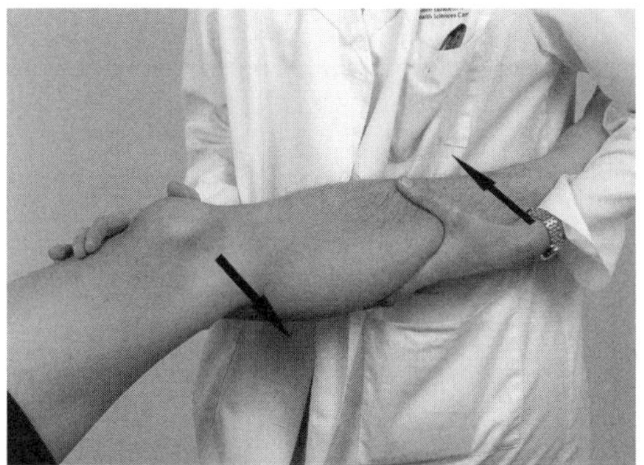

Figure 67. MCL stability test - arrows indicate the direction of forces applied across the knee joint to stress the MCL

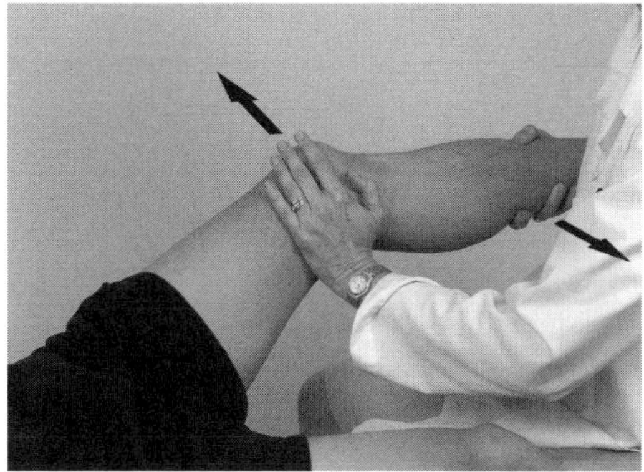

Figure 68. LCL stability test - - arrows indicate the direction of forces applied across the knee joint to stress the LCL

the knee. If a space opens medially it may be visible (called gapping) and when the stress is released you may feel the tibia and femur clunk back into place. If this occurs the medial collateral ligament is significantly torn and it will not support the knee properly (figure 67).

To test the lateral collateral ligament, you will need to 'gap' the knee along its lateral joint line. Use the same technique as for the medial collateral ligament, but reverse the lines of force. That is, apply a varus force through the knee. Grasp the lower leg as described above but with your hands in opposite positions. Simultaneously apply counter forces through the distal medial thigh and the lateral malleolus and observe for gapping (figure 68). When the stress is relieved a clunk may be appreciated if the ligament is completely torn.

Cruciate Ligaments

The anterior and posterior cruciate ligaments are crucial in providing stability to the knee as they control excessive anterior and posterior movement of the femur with respect to the tibia. First, have the patient lie supine and flex their knee to approximately 90°. Stabilize the lower leg by sitting on the patient's foot, then grasp just below the joint line and firmly pull the lower leg towards you (figure 69, next page). If the tibia slides forward from under the femur (a positive *anterior drawer test*) the ACL may be torn. A few degrees of anterior draw are normal if the findings are the same in the opposite knee.

To test the integrity of the posterior cruciate ligament, have the patient in the same position as above but push the tibial plateau posteriorly. If there is significant backward movement, the PCL is probably torn. It is extremely rare to have an isolated tear of the posterior cruciate ligament but not so of the anterior ligament. Remember to do all tests in both knees and compare the findings.

Meniscal Testing

Test for a torn meniscus by bringing different parts of the tibial plateau into contact with the femoral condyle. To test for a medial meniscal tear, narrow the medial compartment of the knee by applying a varus force, then flex and extend the knee while simultaneously internally and externally rotating the tibia.

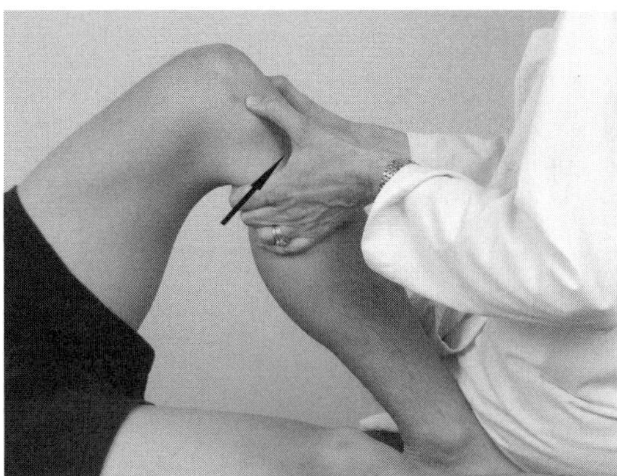

Figure 69. ACL stability test (Anterior Drawer) - the arrow indicates the direction of force applied across the knee joint to stress the ACL. The examiners thumbs palpate for the degree of 'give' betweeen the femur and tibia

To test for lateral meniscal tear, do the same but apply a valgus force to the knee. If a patient becomes markedly apprehensive, experiences pain or if the joint locks, the test is considered positive.

Always remember to keep in mind the patient's complaints. Do the physical exam findings agree with your clinical suspicions? Is the patient complaining of knee pain but the knee exam is normal? If so, you must evaluate the joint above and below (i.e. the hip and ankle) and do a neurologic exam. Lumbar spine pathology may manifest as pain in the knee. *Three to the knee and four to the floor* is a rhyme to help remember the dermatomes of the leg.

Clinical Vignettes

1. *A 36-year-old businessman presents with a complaint of pain, swelling and redness of the right knee. He enjoys good general health and exercises regularly. The pain and swelling developed suddenly yesterday evening and became worse overnight. He has not had any fever or chills, and he otherwise feels well. His gait is not antalgic, but he is very careful as he lifts his pantleg above the knee to avoid the cloth touching the anterior surface of his knee. On examination there is marked redness and swelling over the anterior surface of the knee, directly overlying the patella. The area of redness is very hot and tender to touch. He is able to flex and extend the knee, but with flexion the pain is made slightly worse, and the area of redness becomes well demarcated. You are able to avoid the area of redness and can perform a test looking for a fluid 'bulge' in the medial compartment, but detect none.*

This gentleman has classic pre-patellar septic bursitis. This is not the picture of septic arthritis; the well demarcated area of swelling with knee flexion points to bursal rather than joint swelling. As well, his gait is not antalgic. Pain from septic arthritis is usually severe and patients will limp severely if they can walk at all. The area of redness is well circumscribed and is accentuated by knee flexion because of the increased pressure in the bursa. The appropriate management is aspirating the bursa and sending the fluid for culture. The patient should be started on oral antibiotics. Fortunately, the prepatellar bursa does not usually communicate with the knee joint and septic arthritis is an unlikely but possible consequence. Frequently patients cannot recall any precipitating event for septic bursitis, which may be caused by a break in the skin from a minor abrasion or an insect bite with secondary contamination with bacteria.

2. *A 72 year old man complains of right knee pain of insidious onset. Pain is present with*

weight bearing but it can also be present at rest. He finds it difficult to go from sitting to standing because of pain, and he has had to give up long walks because of the pain. He has not noticed any joint swelling or redness, and although he does experience some left knee discomfort, it does not concern him.

On exam, his gait is antalgic with a decreased stance phase on the right leg. There is no varus or valgus deformity of the knees, and you detect no erythema, increased temperature or joint swelling. Tests for ligamentous stability and integrity of the menisci are normal. None of the maneuvers exacerbate or alleviate his discomfort. When asked to pinpoint exactly where in his knee he feels the pain, he cannot do so, as the 'pain is deep'.

To further sort out this patient's complaints at the bedside, a hip exam is necessary. In this case, he has marked restriction of internal rotation, abduction and adduction of the right hip. He had no groin pain but movement of his hip aggravated his knee pain. Radiographs revealed advanced osteoarthritis of the right hip. Subsequent to hip replacement surgery, his knee pain disappeared.

CHAPTER NINE

Examination of the Ankle

The ankle and foot are usually discussed under one heading, but for purposes of clarity they are discussed separately here. The ankle joint is a simple hinge joint, where the talus articulates with the tibia and the fibula, permitting only two movements, plantar and dorsiflexion, in one plane. Complaints of pain may result from problems within the joint, they may be referred from more proximal regions such as the knee, hip or lumbar spine or they may be secondary to a neurologic problem.

Interestingly, the common term 'sprained ankle' is a misnomer as it is not representative of a true ankle sprain. It is a sprain of the anterior talofibular ligament and most frequently results from excessive inversion at the subtalar joint. However, in more severe cases, the distal anterior tibiofibular ligament can be injured in addition to the anterior talofibular ligament.

Inspection

As with all weight bearing joints the ankle should initially be inspected with the patient standing. Normally the lateral malleolus is closer to the floor than the medial malleolus, but in some conditions, such as rheumatoid arthritis, there may be plantar migration of the medial malleolus. Look for localized or diffuse swelling and for any colour changes. When inspecting the posterior aspect of the ankle, look carefully at the Achilles's tendon for nodules, xanthomas or asymmetry in tendon and muscle bulk. Observe the patient's gait. Is it balanced? Are they able to heel strike and toe-off normally or are there signs of a drop foot? Are they twisting their lower leg sideways to propel themselves forward? Shoes should be examined for patterns of wear (see foot examination for more details).

Palpation

Feel for increased tissue temperature over the anterior surface of the ankle joint and compare to the belly of the calf muscles. Identify the bony landmarks and palpate each of the following: the medial malleolus, lateral malleolus, calcaneus and the dome (top) of the talus. Next, identify the Achilles tendon, anterior talofibular ligament and the deltoid ligament.

The anterior talofibular ligament is not distinctly palpable, but if sprained, there is swelling and tenderness in the sinus tarsi. To appreciate these effusions, invert the patient's foot and palpate between the anterior lateral malleolus and the tarsal bone.

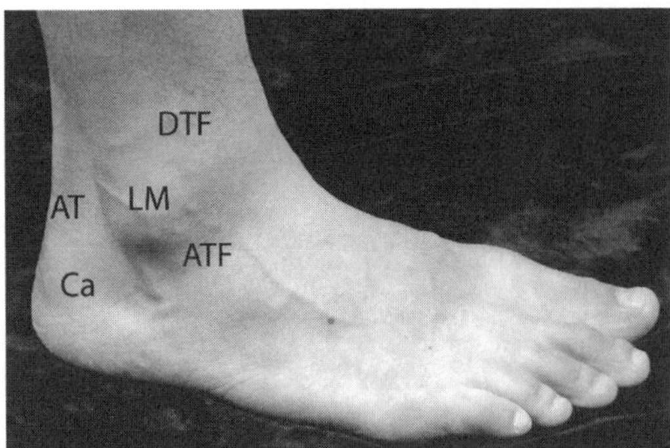

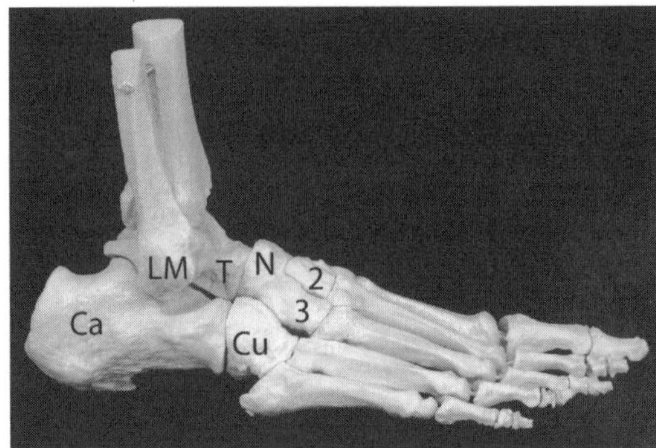

Figure 70A. Surface & Bony Anatomy - Lateral Ankle: DTF - position of distal anterior tibiofibular joint; LM = lateral malleolus; AT = achilles tendon;Ca = calcaneus; ATF = position of anterior talofibular ligament; T = talus; Cu = cuboid; N = navicular; 2 = 2nd cuneiform; 3 = 3rd cuneiform.

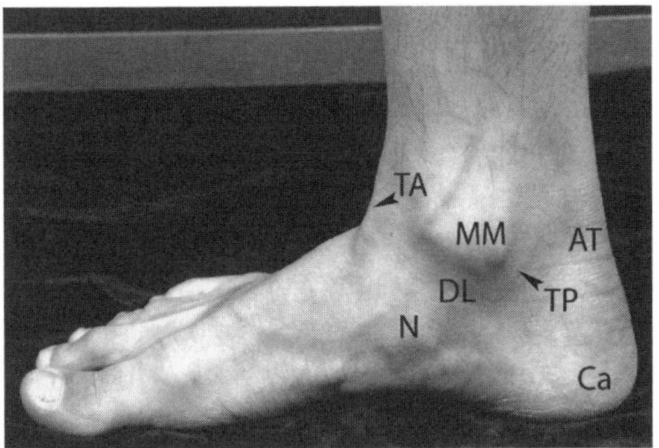

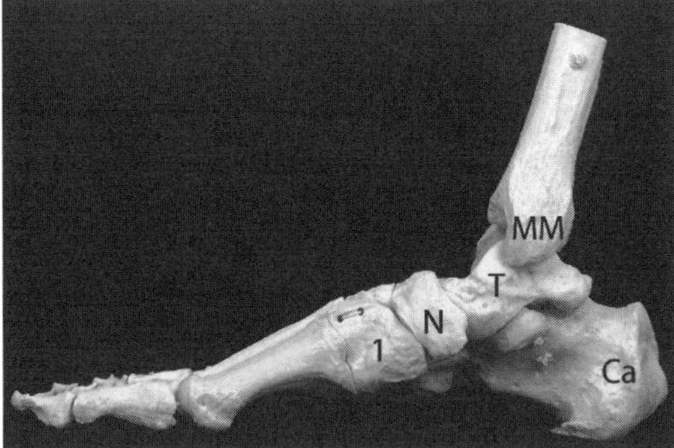

Figure 70B. Surface & Bony Anatomy - Medial Ankle: TA = tibialis anterior tendon; MM = medial malleolus; AT = achilles tendon; TP = tibialis posterior tendon; Ca = calcaneus; DL = deltoid ligament; N = navicular; T = talus; 1 = 1st cuneiform.

Range of Motion

Dorsi and plantar flexion are the only two movements of the ankle joint. The most common mistake students make is in their assessment of dorsi flexion; the knee must be in flexion for proper evaluation. Short gastrocnemius and/or soleus muscles will impede both passive and active dorsiflexion. Many a student and resident, after examining the ankle with the knee straight, has confidently expressed the belief that the ankle cannot be dorsiflexed beyond a 90° angle (the neutral position). Look at your own ankle the next time you descendthe stairs: the trailing foot must be able to dorsiflex at least 20° (from neutral position) to allow you to step down without twisting your body sideways or forcing you to take one step at a time. Patients who have had serious damage to their ankle either through illness or injury may have to navigate steps in this way but it certainly is not normal. Plantar flexion normally is approximately 50° from the foot's neutral position.

Special Tests

Tests for Ankle Joint Stability

The anterior drawer test assesses the integrity of the anterior talofibular ligament. Cup the patient's heel in your hand, stabilize the tibia with your other hand, and draw the heel firmly towards yourself. Normally there is no or very little movement, but if the ligament is

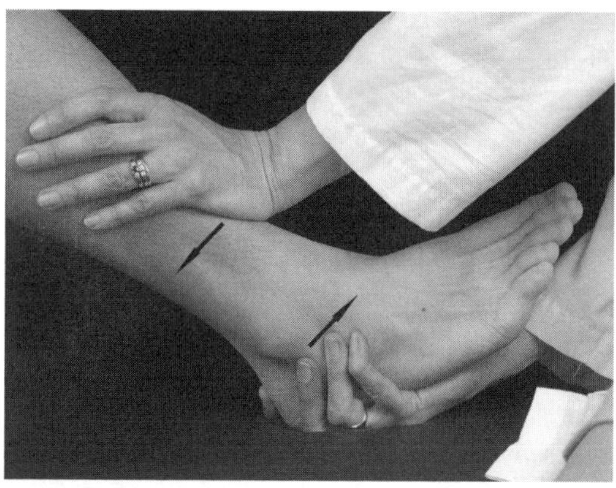

Figure 71. Anterior drawer test for the ankle - arrows indicate the direction of forces applied across the ankle to stress the anterior talofibular ligament.

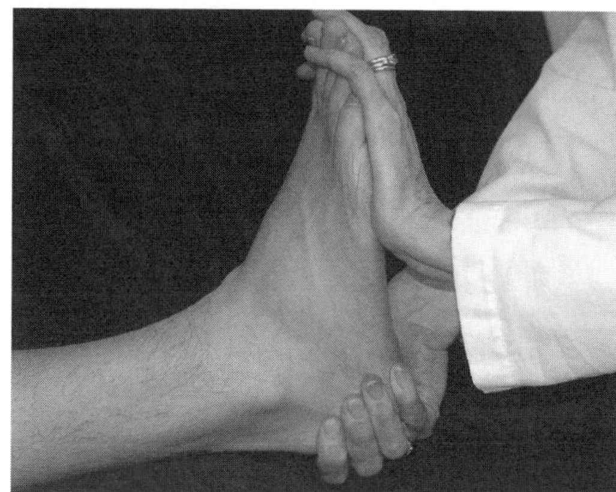

Figure 73. Subtalar joint stability test.

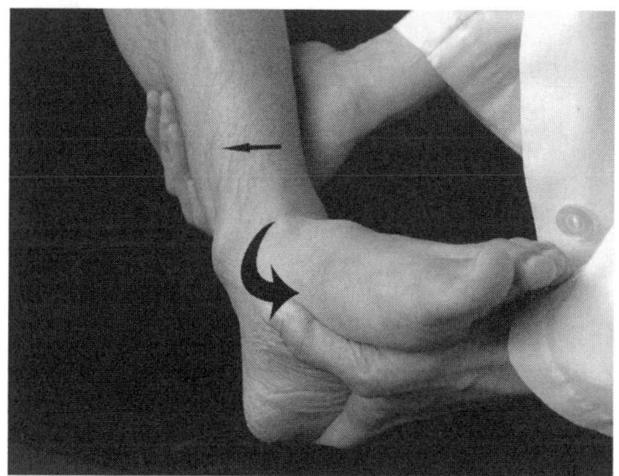

Figure 72. Test of the medial collateral ligament (deltoid ligament) - arrows indicate the forces applied across the subtalar joint to stress the deltoid ligament.

disrupted the talus will slide forwards and you may even feel a 'clunk' (figure 71).

To test lateral and medial stability of the ankle, keep the ankle in a neutral position and apply pressure to invert and evert the calcaneus relative to the talus. Cupping the heel (the calcaneus) while keeping the ankle in neutral allows you to apply pressure in the appropriate direction (figure 72).

The subtalar complex is actually made up of three joints: the posterior talocalcanean, the talo-calcaneo-navicular and the transverse tarsal joints. For examination purposes they are assessed as one. With one hand maintain the ankle joint in full dorsiflexion. With the other hand cupping the heel, apply inversion and eversion forces through the subtalar joint; there should be only 3-5 degrees of movement (figure 73).

A detailed discussion of the individual ligaments and tendons that cross the ankle is not in the mandate of this summary, but the interested student is encouraged to read *Physical Examination of the Spine and Extremities* by Stanley Hoppenfeld. However, if you can remember your basic anatomy, you need not memorize any special tests. To test ligaments, passively stretch them along their long axis. For questions of tendinitis, place the tendon under either a stretch or a stress. If a tendon is torn, the clinician will be unable to stretch it or stress it: Can you think what you might see if the Achilles tendon was torn?

Clinical Hint:

Think of its primary function, i.e. to plantar flex the foot. If it is torn, do you think the gait would be normal? Would the patient be able to stand on their toes? If it is torn, what happens to the muscle attached to the tendon? Would you expect to see anything unusual at the site of attachment? The foot exam naturally flows from the ankle and sub-talar exams and in clinical practice one would not examine one without the other.

Clinical Vignettes

1. *A 23-year-old woman presents with severe bilateral ankle pain and swelling. Onset dates to approximately ten days ago. Initially she noted swelling and redness in her right ankle but within two days her left ankle was also involved. She is able to walk, but as the day progresses the pain and swelling intensify.*

On examination there is marked redness over both medial malleoli, extending to the anterior surface of the joint, and non-tender swelling is present posteriorly in the region of the Achilles tendons. Palpation does reveal the ankles to be tender and warm, but there is full range of motion in both ankles, and pain is exacerbated not by movement but with weight bearing.

This can be a perplexing presentation. The first question the clinician must address is whether this young woman has true ankle joint effusions or whether this is a 'peri-arthropathy', a problem around but not within the joint. The physical exam suggests that the problem is not within the joint because she has painfree movement of the joint. The increased pain upon weight bearing is non-specific and may be due to increased blood flow and increased oncotic pressure. The marked redness of skin also points away from a true synovitis; gout can cause marked redness of skin but most inflammatory arthropathies do not (gout is not a tenable diagnosis in a young woman except in very rare cases). The erythema, local tenderness, surrounding edema and normal movement of the ankles are in keeping with erythema nodosum, an inflammatory process in the subcutaneous tissues (panniculitis). This, in itself, is not a diagnosis as erythema nodosum can be associated with a number of conditions including, but not limited to, inflammatory bowel disease, strep throat infection, birth control pills, some antibiotics, and a condition called sarcoidosis. Of course, it may occur without a known cause,which case it is termed 'idiopathic'. The bottom line is that just because a joint looks swollen does not mean that it is. Use all your clinical skills, temper them with experience and knowledge, and you can solve the problem and help your patient.

2. *A 19-year-old college student complains of a two-week history of painful swelling in his right ankle. He does not recall injuring it but he figures he must have hurt it playing soccer a few weeks ago. He has been otherwise well, and denies any other health concerns. He is unaware of any family history of arthritis.*

On examination, there is marked swelling of the right Achilles tendon. It is tender to palpation and dorsiflexion of the ankle is restricted because of pain in the ankle. The remainder of the examination is unremarkable except for the presence of nail pits in the second and third fingers of his right hand and the fourth finger of his left hand, and some red scaling skin around his umbilicus.

This young man has Achilles tendonitis. The presence of nail pits and the peri-umbilical redness and scaling of skin are suggestive of psoriasis. He most likely has early psoriatic arthritis, with tendonitis being his initial presentation.

CHAPTER TEN

Examination of the Foot

Inspection

Feet ruin shoes, not vice versa, hence the recommendation to begin the examination of the foot by examining the patient's footwear. Look for asymmetry of wear at the heels, examine the creases in the shoes and search for seams which may be parting. Watch the patient walking with their shoes on and off. Are compensatory maneuvers present? Just as in the hand examination, much can be gleaned about the patient's general health from inspection of the feet. Is there cyanosis, mottling of the skin, or signs of chronic poor hygiene? Look at the toenails: is there pitting, marked thickness of the nails or signs of ingrown toenails? It may sound obvious, but count the toes; anything other than the usual ten should be noted (if for no other reason, the patient will notice if the clinician doesn't take note of their unusual allotment of digits).

Foot deformities may be congenital or acquired. Make note of the relative size of the two feet; a marked difference may reflect a repaired congenital deformity such as a clubfoot. Evaluate the arch of the foot. The medial border of the foot should not be so low as to touch the floor or to lift the lateral border of the foot off the floor. Draw an imaginary line from the medial heel toward the great toe to assess for hallux valgus (remember the 'L' in valgus is for lateral deviation) or metatarsus varus deformities. The soles of the feet should be examined, and note made of calluses or plantar warts. Deformities of toes should be noted.

Palpation

Start by checking for increased temperature over the midfoot and at the base of the MTP joints. Gently palpate each MTP and IP joint for tenderness and for swelling, using the same four finger technique used in palpating the finger joints (see page 6).

Identify the following bony landmarks and check for tenderness and swelling; the calcaneus, the navicular, and the first through fifth metatarsal bones. Make note of callus and bunion formation if present.

Range of Motion

Active

First do a general screening of the patient's active range of motion. Ask the patient to walk on their toes, then their heels, on the lateral borders of their feet and on the medial borders of their feet. This tests more than just range of motion, of course, but it serves as a good quick test for major problems with the feet and ankles. If there is limitation of

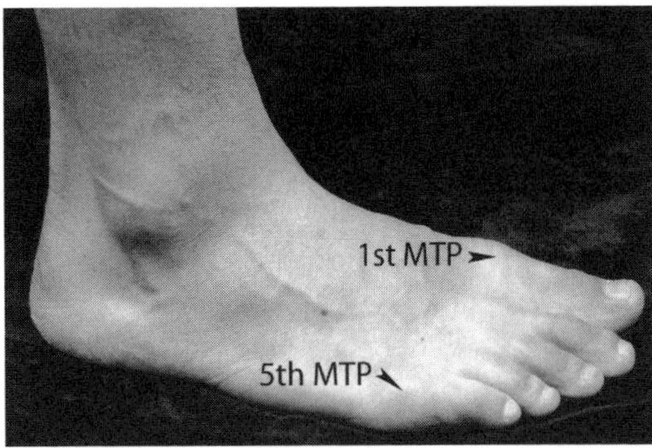

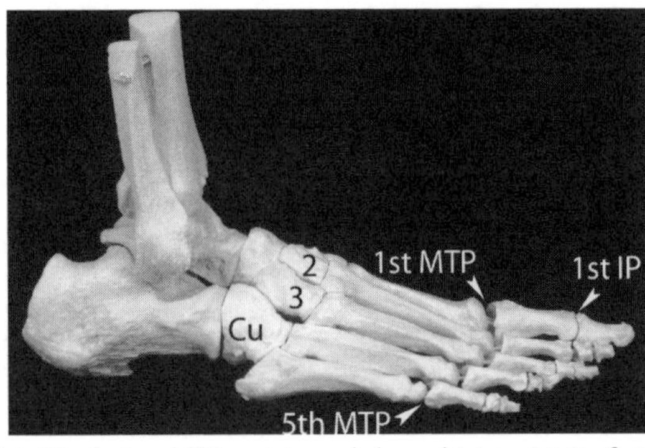

Figure 74A. Surface & Bony Anatomy - Lateral Foot: 1st MTP & 5th MTP = first and fifth metatarsophalangeal joints; 1st IP = first interphalangeal joint; Cu = cuboid; 3 = 3rd cuneiform; 2 = 2nd cuneiform.

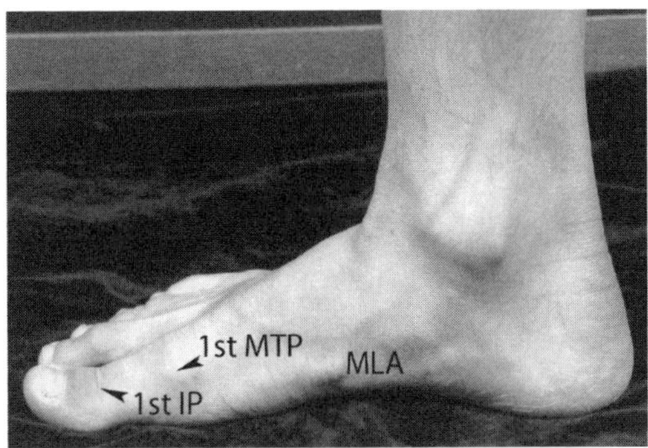

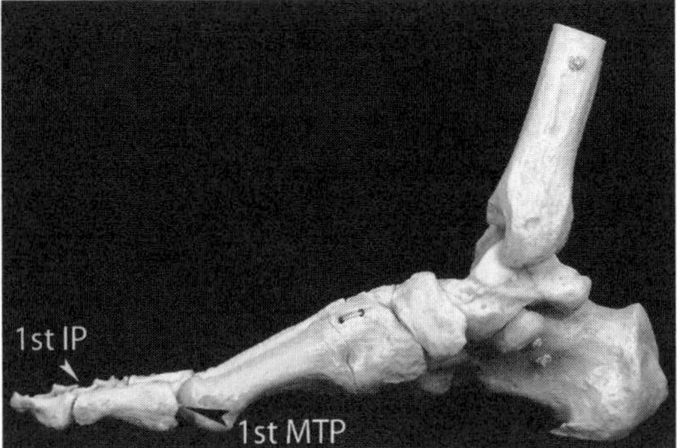

Figure 74B. Surface & Bony Anatomy - Medial Foot: 1st MTP = first metatarsophalangeal joint; 1st IP = first interphalangeal joint; MLA = medial longitudinal arch (partially formed by the plantar fascia).

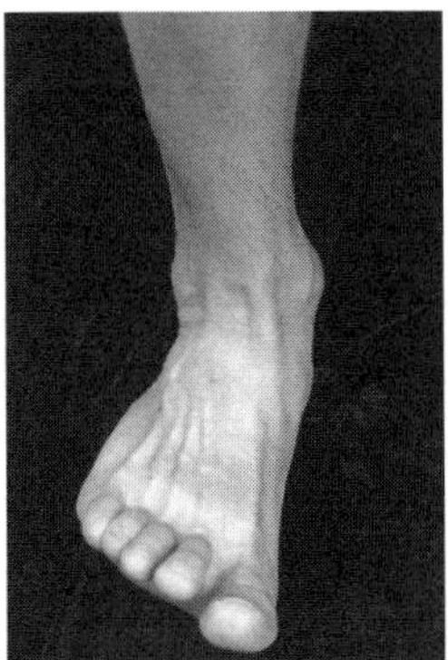

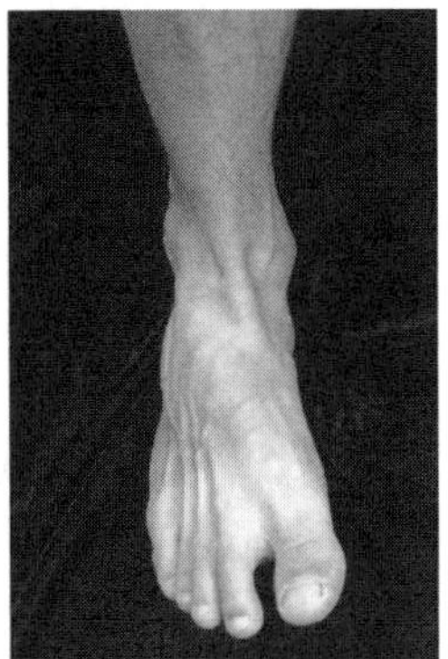

Figure 75 A & B. Left - active eversion; Right - active inversion.

motion, passive range of motion testing is required.

Passive

In the foot, passive movement tests may be performed at the subtalar joint, the forefoot joints or the joints of the digits or toes.

Subtalar Joint: Inversion and Eversion

The subtalar joint actually comprises three joints: the talocalcaneal, the talonavicular and the calcaneocuboid joints. Inversion and eversion occur at these joints and allows one to walk on uneven ground. To test, have the patient's ankle in neutral position, grasp the heel (the calcaneus) and invert and evert the subtalar joint. Normal range is approximately 5°. Pain and/or loss of mobility with this maneuver may be secondary to trauma or arthritis. *Forefoot: Adduction, Abduction, Inversion and Eversion*

Most forefoot movement occurs at the talonavicular and calcaneocuboid joints. Hold the ankle in neutral position to stabilize it and move the forefoot medially and laterally to evaluate adduction and abduction. The movement is more easily felt than seen. For inversion and eversion, grasp the forefoot and rotate it about the long axis of the foot.

Toes: Flexion and Extension

Extension of the first MTP joint is crucial in the 'pre-swing' phase of a normal gait; a minimum of 35-40° extension is required, but the normal toe will move 70-90°. Assess this by stabilizing the foot, then flexing and extending the toe at the MTP joint. The IP joint of the great toe is capable of flexion and essentially has no extension.

The second through fifth toes should be assessed for flexion and extension at the MTP, PIP and DIP joints. For normal walking extension at the MTP joints is important. Flexion is utilized during the stance phase of walking for extra stability, especially when walking on uneven ground such as sand.

Special Tests

Plantar Fasciitis

Inflammation of the plantar fascia may result from mechanical imbalances of the lower leg and foot or be associated with a seronegative inflammatory arthritis. Pain is usually felt in the heel and the proximal sole.

As a test, cup the heel with your hand and firmly squeeze the calcaneus. If the fascia is inflamed the patient will complain of pain. Putting the fascia under a stretch is another test for plantar fasciitis and is accomplishedby stabilizing the ankle joint and passively extending the forefoot and MTP joints, again looking for complaints of pain (figure 76).

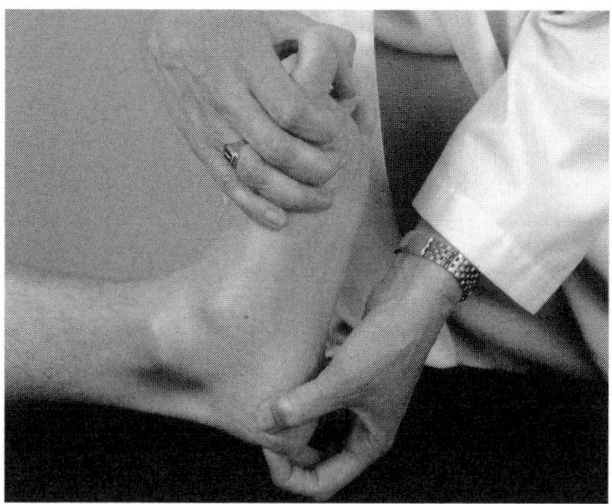

Figure 76. Testing for plantar fasciitis.

Clinical Vignettes

1. *A 33 year old woman presents with complaints of painful feet. She has been experiencing difficulties finding comfortable footwear because of pain at the base of her toes. She cannot recall when her symptoms started, but they have been present for the past two or three months. She has been feeling well otherwise. She has no other health concerns and her past medical history has been unremarkeale.*

On examination her gait is antalgic. She pivots her entire foot to avoid the toe-off phase of walking. Inspection of her feet while she is standing reveals splaying of the second and third toes bilaterally and the patient remarks on this being new for her. There is tenderness across the MTP joints with gentle squeezing of the forefoot; individually, all the MTP joints are tender to palpation. Your are not sure, but you think the second and third MTP joints are swollen. The rest of the foot examination is normal.

You can trust your fingers. The joints are swollen in this scenario; the splaying of the toes is the sure-fire sign of MTP joint swelling, especially when the patient tells you her feet never looked like that before. This young woman has inflammatory arthritis, and she needs further diagnostic workup.

2. *A 55-year-old woman complains of marked pain in the great toes of both feet. They do not pain when she wears low-heeled shoes, but while wearing dress shoes, her feet ache terrifically. She is unaware of swelling, but she has been dismayed by how 'old' her feet look.*

On examination her gait is not antalgic and her footwear today is a comfortable pair of soft leather walking shoes. There is marked hallux valgus of both feet, but range of motion in the MTP joints is preserved. The great toes are mildly tender to palpation. The rest of the examination is normal.

This woman has osteoarthritis of the first MTP joints bilaterally - you do not need a radiograph to make the diagnosis. She should be encouraged to continue to wear low-heeled shoes. Surgery is an option, but should be reserved for when she can no longer find comfortable footwear.

CHAPTER ELEVEN

A Screening Exam

The preceding chapters hopefully will have provided you with the necessary knowledge and with practice, the skills to evaluate single or regional joint complaints. But how does one assess patients with diffuse aches and pains? Are they among the "worried well" or are their complaints representative of an inflammatory arthropathy? The busy clinician needs an efficient and accurate screening physical examination to complement the history, and to assist in determining whether more detailed examination and investigations are warranted.

Fortunately, clinician-researchers in Britain have developed just such a tool and labeled it the 'GALS locomotor screen'. No, it is not a screen for women only, but rather a mnemonic for Gait, Arms, Legs and Spine. Although initially tested and validated in an inpatient hospital unit, it has since been proven accurate and sensitive in outpatient adult and pediatric populations. A screening tool by necessity will not incorporate all that is required of a detailed examination, so you should not be surprised that this screen relies primarily on a brief history followed by inspection, range of motion, some palpation, and that there are no 'special tests'.

History

In the first chapter the importance of the history was discussed. Ask the detailed questions if any of the following are answered with a "yes":

1. Do you have any stiffness in your muscles, joints or back?
2. Can you dress yourself completely, without any difficulty?
3. Can you walk up and downstairs without any difficulty?

Physical Examination

Inspection, Palpation and Range of Motion are intermixed!

The patient should be in their underwear or equivalent, and just as with the regional exams, more than one view is required. Although there are several components to the exam, the order in which you do them is not important. Do them in order of what feels most natural to you; a simple checklist will summarize your findings and aid in the interpretation.

Gait: Is there symmetry and smoothness of movement; is the stride length & mechanics of the gait within normal limits; does the patient have the ability to turn quickly?

Standing: While the patient is standing, observe from the back looking for scoliosis, that the iliac crests are level, that the paraspinal muscles are normal, and that there is normal symmetrical muscle bulk of the:

- Shoulders
- Buttocks
- Thighs & calves

Check for absence of swelling in the popliteal and hindfoot regions, and that there is no hindfoot deformity.

From the side, look for normal cervical & lumbar lordosis, and thoracic kyphosis (figure 77). Ask the patient to touch their toes, and observe for normal lumbosacral rhythm.

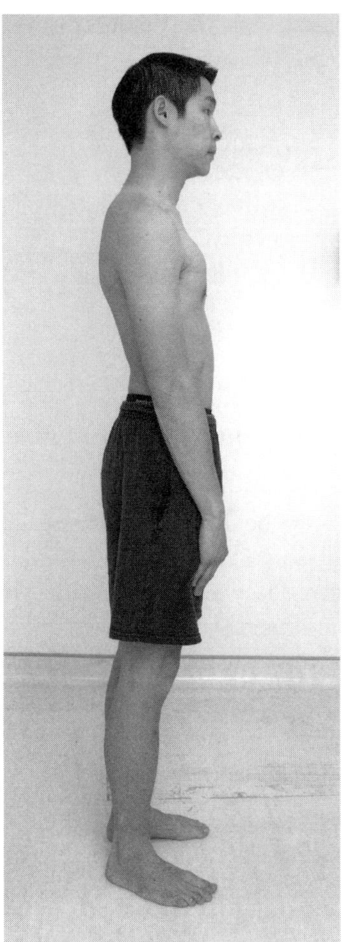

Figure 77. thoracic kyphosis and lumbar lotdosis

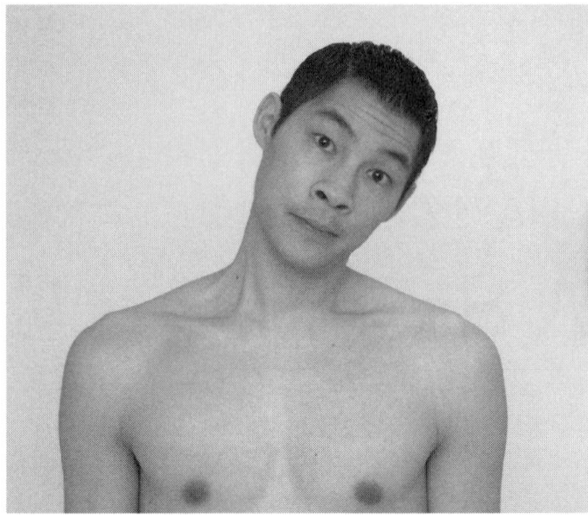

Figure 78. Ear to shoulder

Inspecting from the front, ask the patient to put their ear against their shoulder and then back to neutral (figure 78). Make note of the **Arms:** ask them to bring their:

- 'Arms behind head, elbows back' (figure 79)
- 'Hands down by sides, elbows straight'
- 'Hands in front, palms down' (figure 80)
- 'Turn hands over' (figure 81)
- 'Make a fist'
- 'Fingers on thumb' (figure 83)
- Examiner squeezes metacarpals 2 to 5

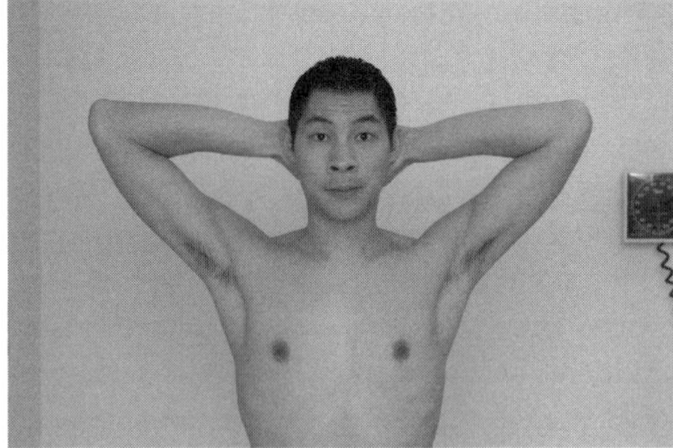

Figure 79. Arms behind head, elbows back

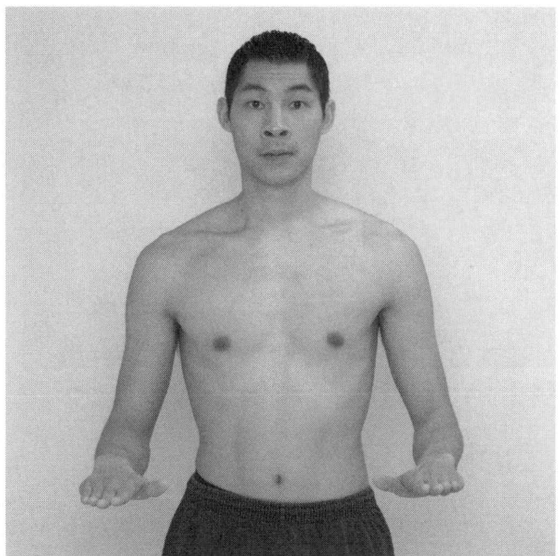

Figure 80. Hands in front, palms down

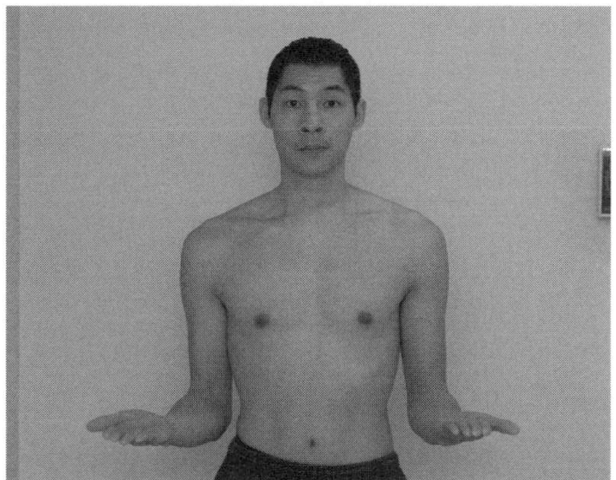

Figure 81. Turn hands over

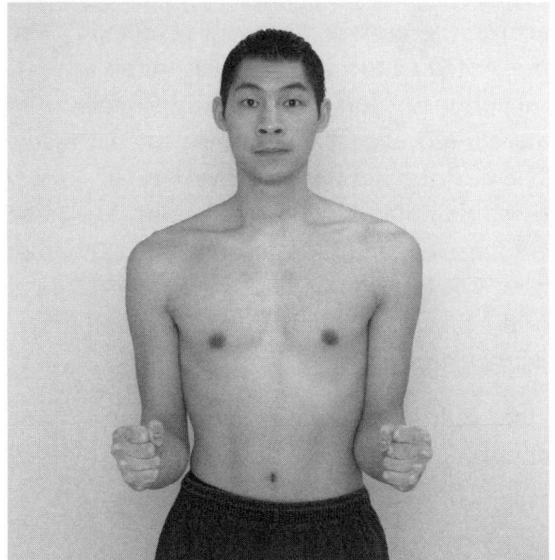

Figure 82.. Make a fist

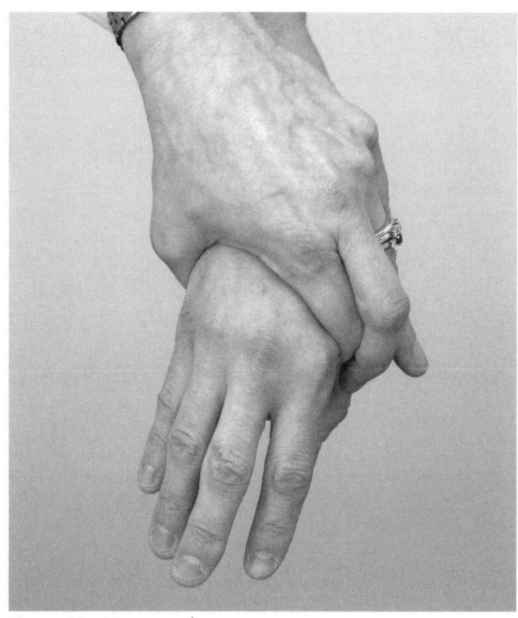

Figure 83. Metacarpal squeeze

Still inspecting from the front, make note of the Legs

- Normal quadriceps bulk & symmetry
- No knee swelling
- No knee valgus or varus
- No forefoot or midfoot deformity
- Normal arches of feet

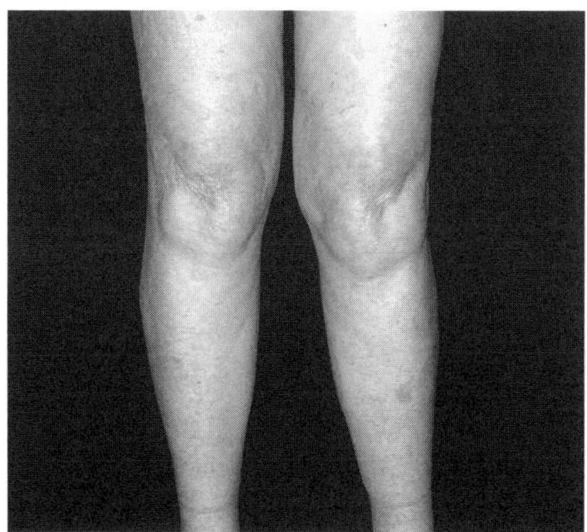

Figure 84. Inspection of Legs
(Note valgus deformity - L leg)

In bed

- Passively flex each hip & knee
  - Knee crepitus??
- Passively internally rotate each hip (figure 85)
- Press on patella
  - Patello-femoral tenderness
  - Knee effusion
- Squeeze metatarsals (figure 86)
- Inspect soles of feet for calluses (figure 87)

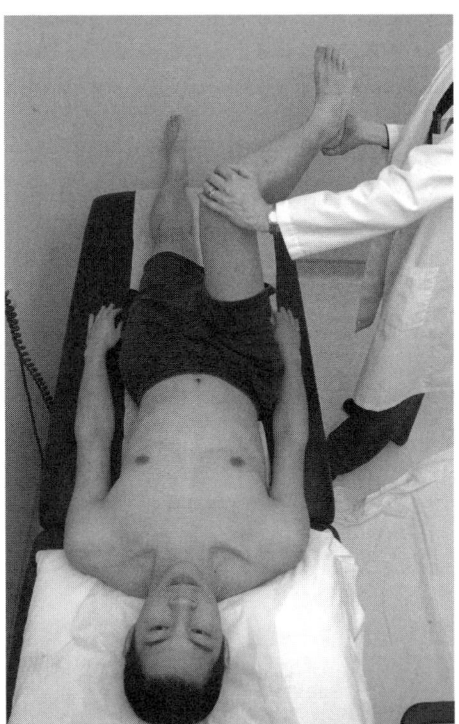

Figure 85. R hip internal rotation

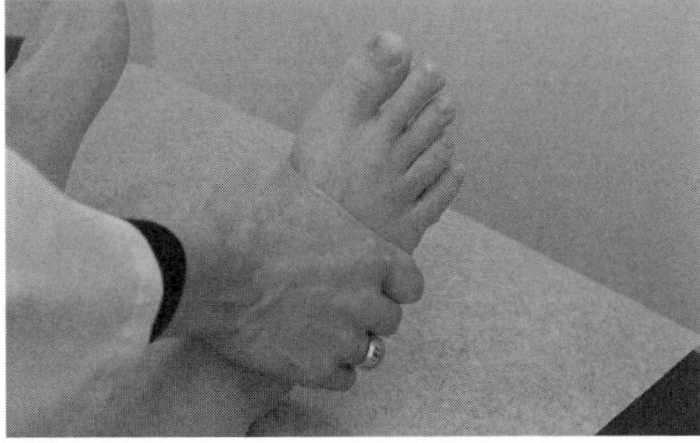

Figure 86. Metatarsal squeeze

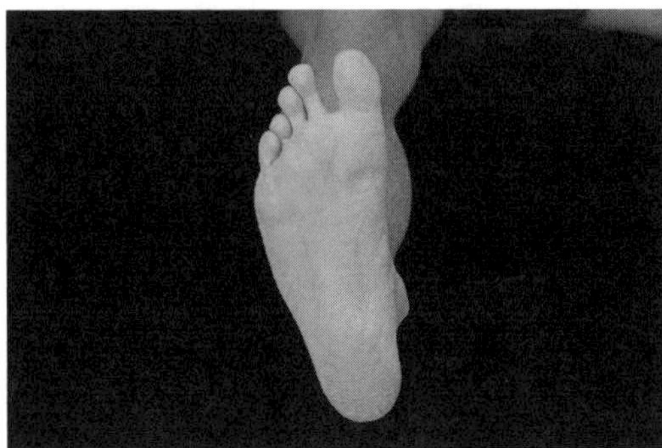

Figure 87. Inspection Bola

Clinical Vignettes

1. *A 45 year old man is concerned about increasing joint stiffness and pain in multiple joints. There is something sore almost every day, including his knees, feet, fingers and hips. Joints feel swollen on occasion and morning stiffness is present for "about 30 minutes". He is particularly worried as his mother suffered from rheumatoid arthritis. He is able to dress himself without any difficulty, and is able to walk up and down stairs but does experience pain in both knees going down stairs.*

The GALS exam reveals no abnormalities except for crepitus in both patellar femoral joints.

This is the perfect scenario for a screening musculoskeletal examination. The patient is at increased risk for developing rheumatoid arthritis because of his family history, and the presence of morning stiffness, although not exceptionally long, is still a bit longer than one would expect in primary osteoarthritis. The GALS exam has effectively ruled out active inflammatory joint disease; he does have evidence of patello-femoral crepitus and may have OA of the patello-femoral joint; x-rays of the knees will confirm and physiotherapy may be appropriate.

One could record the findings using "+" for abnormal and "√" for normal, i.e.:

History: Pain + *
Dress √
Walk √

*diffuse pain, knees in particular with descending stairs

G √	Appearance	Movement
A	√	√
L	√	+ *
S	√	√

* crepitus both patellofemoral joints

2. *A 33year old woman is 4 months postpartum and she has been feeling miserable with poor energy but she blames this on being awakened frequently by her newborn. She has not been able to lose weight since the birth of the baby.*

This is another appropriate scenario for the GALS.

The three screening questions:

1. **Have you any pain or stiffness in your muscles, joints or back?**
   She replies that her fingers and feet have been sore.
2. **Can you dress yourself completely without difficulty?**
   Small buttons and zippers are difficult because her fingers are very stiff and sore, especially in the morning.
3. **Can you walk up and down stairs without difficulty?**
   Her feet are so sore that she has to take one step at a time. She has been blaming the extra weight on making her feet sore.

   The physical examination reveals an antalgic gait and pain in the MCP and MTP joints when pressure is applied across the metacarpals and metatarsals respectively.

   The findings on history and physical are recorded:

   Pain + fingers and feet
   Dress + *buttons and zippers*
   Walk + metatarsalgia

G +	Appearance	Movement
A	+	+
L	√	+
S	√	√

Gait: avoids toe-off
MCPs appear swollen
Decreased grip
Pain with squeezing hands and feet
Gait antalgic

The screening history and physical are positive and more detailed history and physical examinations are required! There is no question that this young woman is not just suffering from too much "baby weight". The hands and feet require more careful evaluation followed by screening bloodwork for thyroid disease, rheumatoid arthritis and systemic lupus, the 3 most common causes of persistent post-partum joint swelling.

Appendices

Appendix 1.1

Selected Abnormalities of the Articular System

If you are a medical student, allied health professional, post-graduate medical trainee or family physician, confidence in your examination of the musculoskeletal system will serve you well in your profession. The ability to separate inflammatory from non-inflammatory joint disease by history and physical examination allows for appropriate management and utilization of resources. As you can see from the preceding chapters, the MSK exam is neither conceptually nor physically difficult. However, it does require practice to establish confidence in one's own abilities to detect a swollen joint from one that is enlarged by excess bone production. Recognition of visible abnormalities is key to the inspection component of the exam, and in this concluding chapter, some common findings are presented.

1.11 Hand & Wrist

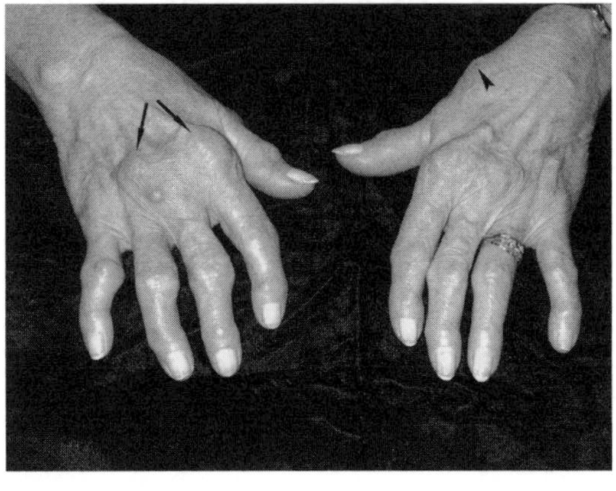

Figure 88. These hands demonstrate both inflammatory and degenerative changes. Note squaring of the left thumb CMC joint (arrow head) and the osteoarthritic changes of the DIP and PIP joints, called Heberden's and Bouchard's nodes respectively. There is no difference in the histopathology; both Heberden's and Bouchard's nodes represent osteophytes at the DIP and PIP joints respectively. This patient also has swelling of the right 2nd and 3rd MCP joints (arrows); she has rheumatoid arthritis superimposed on osteoarthritis.

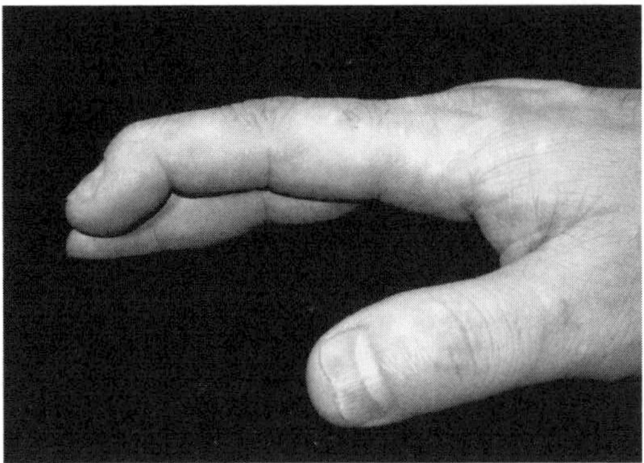

Figure 89. This is a classic mallet finger deformity. The extensor tendon to the DIP joint is disrupted, either from an avulsion injury (as sustained in sports such as softball or basketball) or from fraying and rupture of the tendon from inflammatory arthritis, in this case, psoriatic arthritis. The thumb nail changes are characteristic of psoriatic arthritis.

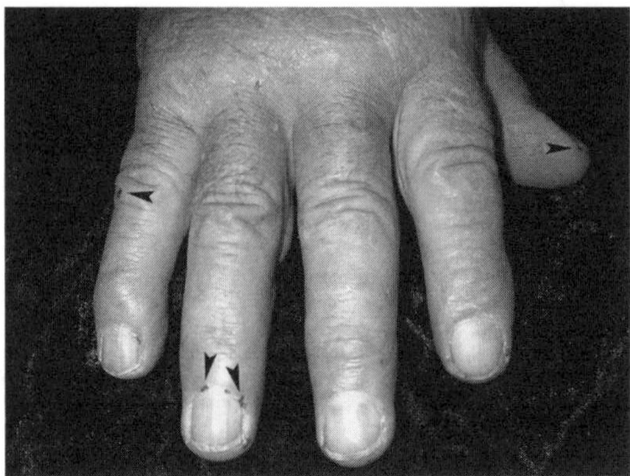

Figure 90. This patient has obvious swelling of the MCP joints, but notice the small lesions indicated by the arrowheads; these are vasculitic lesions. The patient has rheumatoid arthritis, and the lesions could easily be overlooked, but should not be; they are a sign of rheumatoid vasculitis and may portend more serious complications.

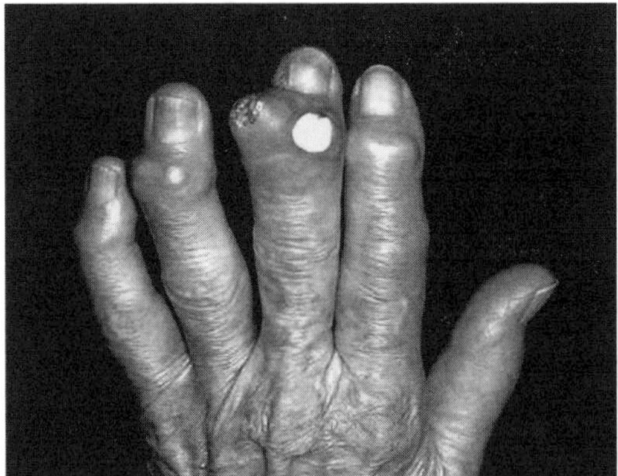

Figure 91A. This woman has terrible swelling, redness and white discharge from her DIP joints. She has tophaceous gout. This is a problem that is joint based, but causes destruction of tissue and bone. See her x-ray in figure 80B.

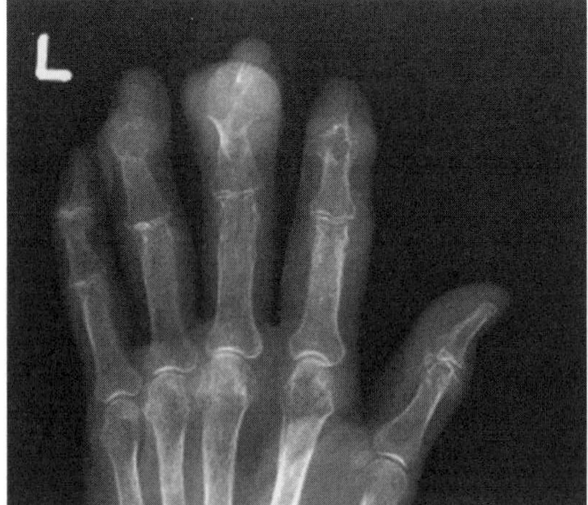

Figure 91B. Note the complete destruction of bone in the 3rd DIP joint. Surprisingly this woman still plays the organ in her local church.

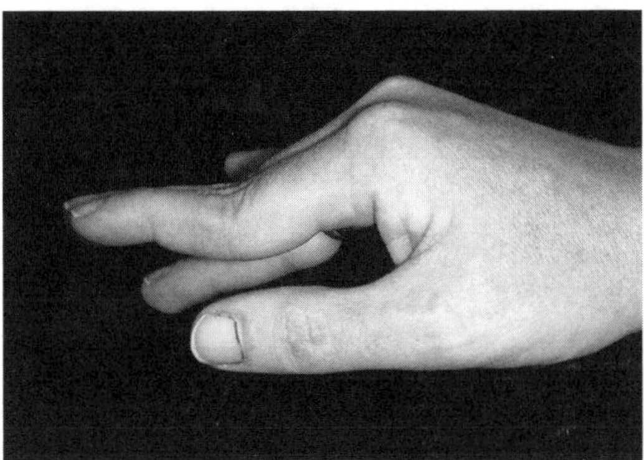

Figure 92. Flexion of the DIP, hyperextension of the PIP and flexion of the MCP joint characterize the Swan Neck deformity. This can be seen in both rheumatoid arthritis and systemic lupus erythematosus. The difference is that the deformity may be reducible in the lupus patient, but it is not in the rheumatoid.

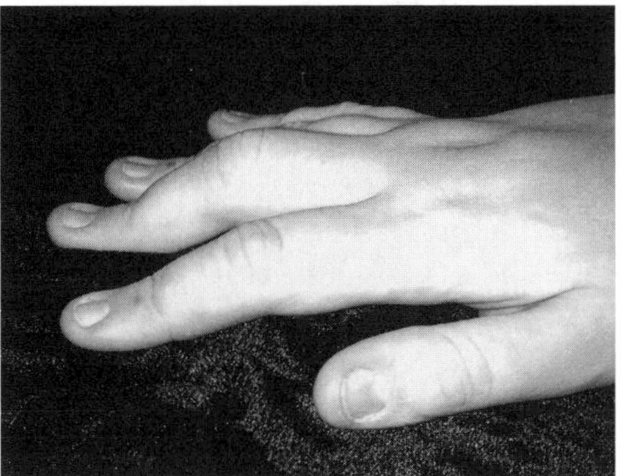

Figure 93. There is marked swelling of the 3rd PIP joint and hyperextension of the DIP joint in keeping with a Boutonniere deformity. This woman has rheumatoid arthritis, but the deformity is also seen frequently in psoriatic arthritis. It is caused by disruption of the PIP volar plate with slippage of the extensor tendons to either side of the joint. The DIP joint is 'pulled' proximally, resulting in the flexed posture of the PIP.

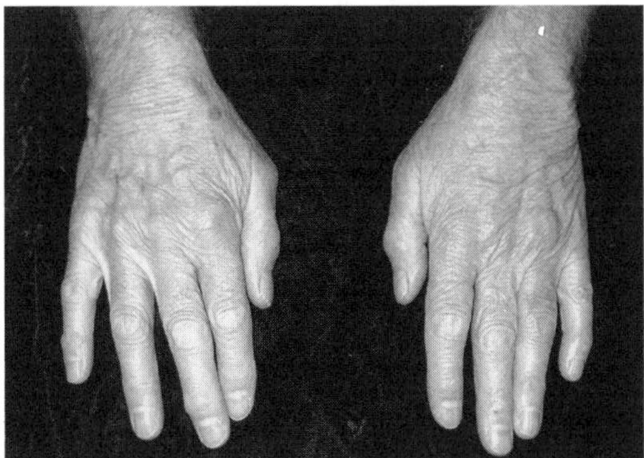

Figure 94A. Inspection is an important part of the wrist examination, but if you relied on this 'bird's eye view' alone, you would miss the significant volar subluxation of the left radio-carpal joint.

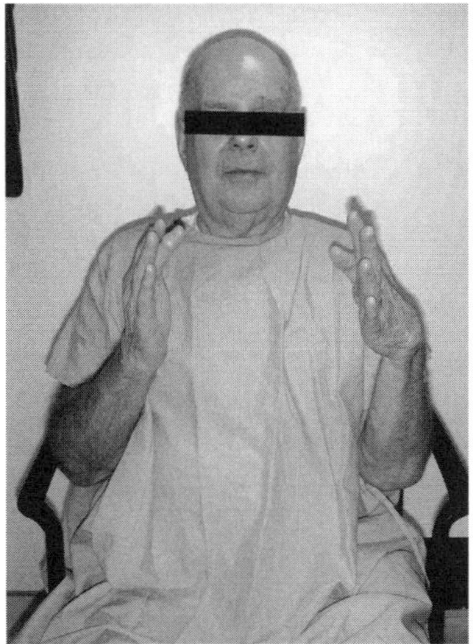

Figure 94B. This gentleman's wrists looked reasonably benign in figure 81A, but this view emphasizes the importance of getting an ulnar view of the wrists.

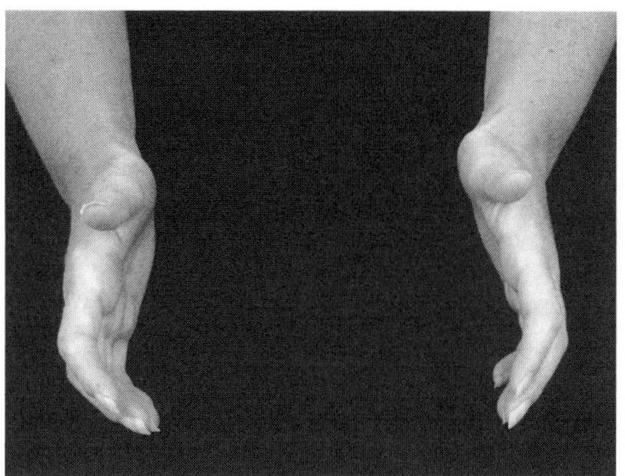

Figure 95A. Observing active range of motion is an important part of the examination. This patient is actively trying to extend her fingers, but she cannot, due to tightness of the skin overlying the joints.

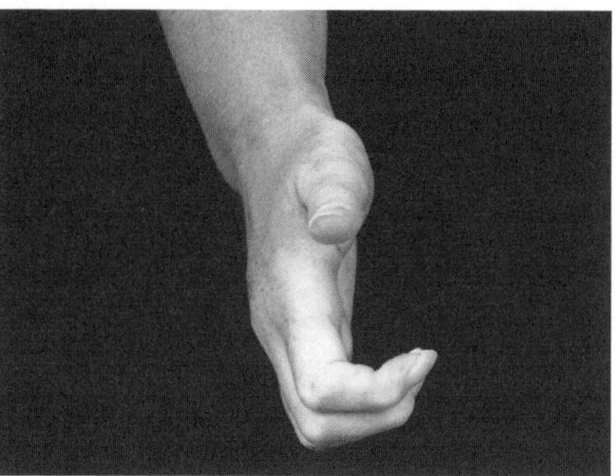

Figure 95B. The same patient tries to demonstrate a finger tuck, but the tightness of her skin prevents further movement.

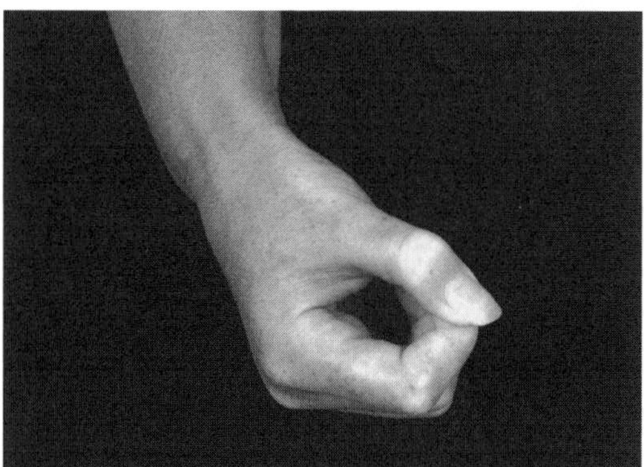

Figure 95C. Finger grip is also restricted. Her joints are pristine, but she has a poor grip because of the marked tightness of the skin secondary to scleroderma.

1.12 Elbow

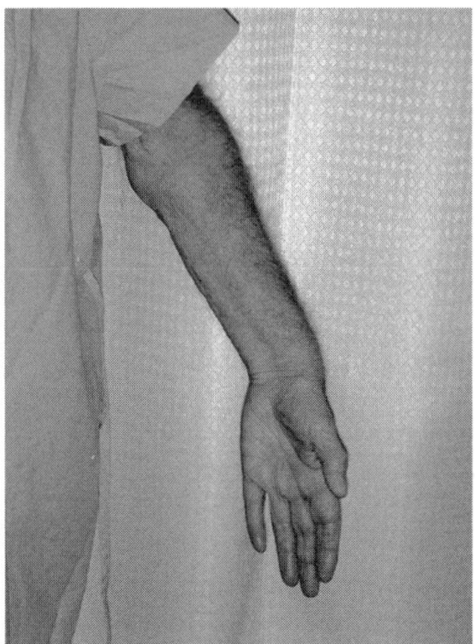

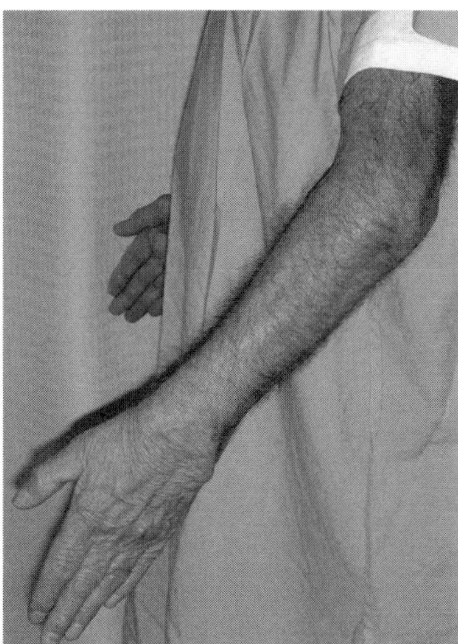

Figure 96. The frontal view suggests a varus deformity of the elbows, but on lateral inspection, a flexion contracture is evident. These photos emphasize the need for inspecting the joints in more than one plane.

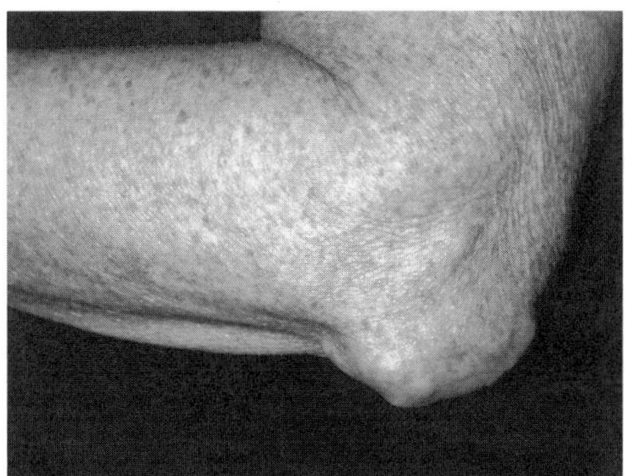

Figure 97. The olecranon bursa is distended with multiple nodules. This can be seen in rheumatoid arthritis and gout.

1.13 Lower Extremity

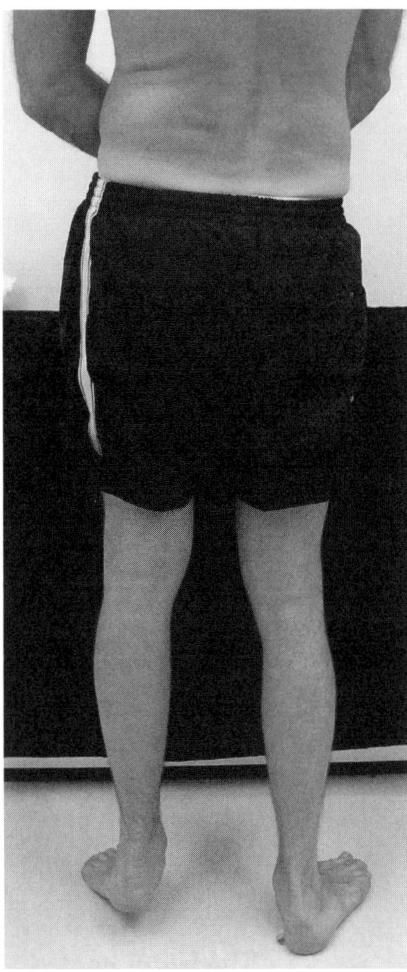

Figure 98A. Leg length discrepancy. This patient is more comfortable with the left ankle in some amount of plantar flexion as evident in the above photograph. Although the patient has bilateral ankle deformities, the cause of the leg length discrepancy is apparent in the hip x-rays (85B). He has severe rheumatoid arthritis of multiple joints, complicated by avascular necrosis secondary to steroid use.

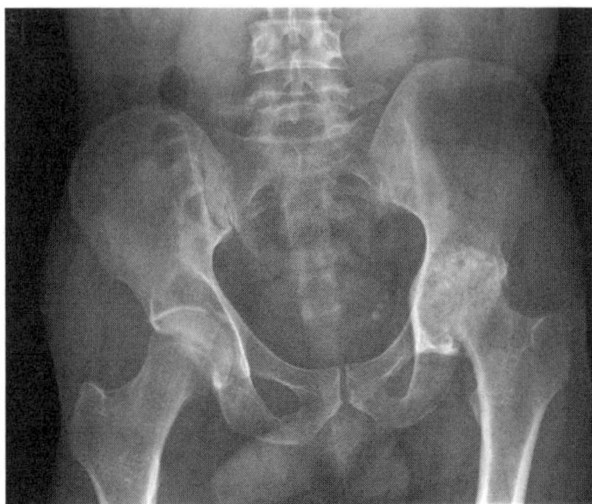

Figure 98B. There is marked joint space narrowing of the left hip, but in addition, the acetabulum is protruding into the pelvic space, hence the term 'acetabulo protrusio'.

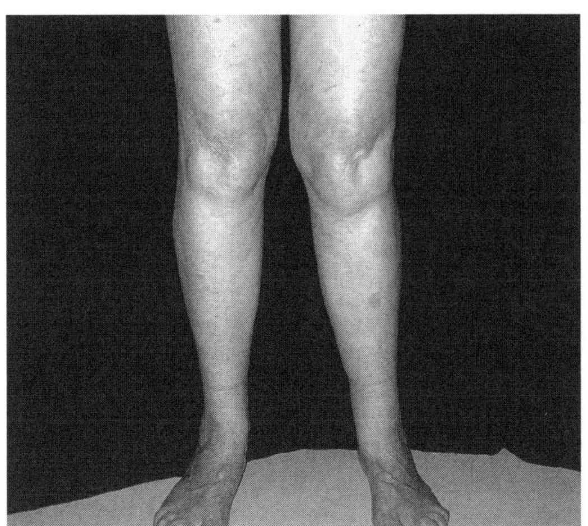

Figure 99. Weight bearing views of the knees should be a mandatory component of inspection, otherwise it would be easy to miss the valgus deformity of this left knee.

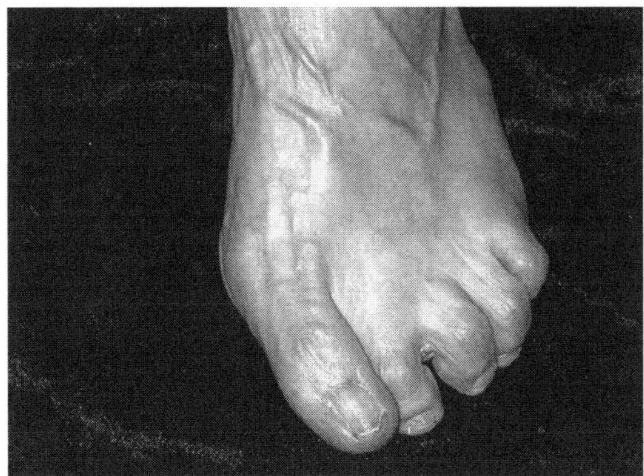

Figure 100. Mild hallux valgus deformity is unlikely to cause this patient discomfort, but the hammer toe deformities of the 2nd through fifth toes will make finding comfortable shoes difficult.

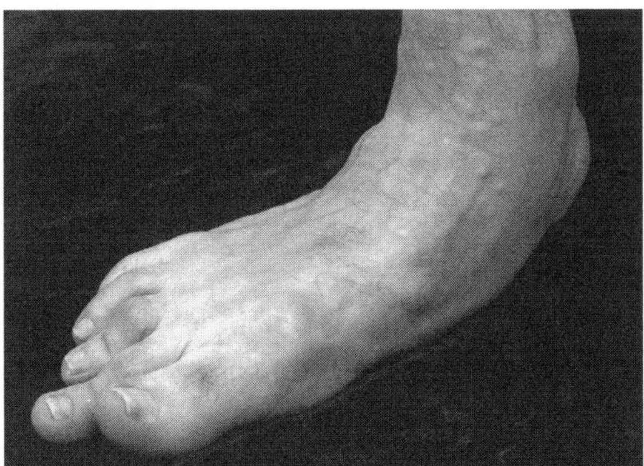

Figure 101. There is complete collapse of the longitudinal arch of the foot secondary to rheumatoid arthritis.

Appendix 1.2

Normal AROM For the Peripheral Joints

Joint	Motion	Range (Degrees)
Finger DIPs	Flexion	0 - 90
	Extension	0 - 10/20
Finger PIPs	Flexion	0 - 110
	Extension	0
Finger MCPs	Flexion	0 - 90
	Extension	0 - 30/45
	Abd/Add	0 - 20
Thumb IP	Flexion	0 - 90
	Extension	0 - 20
Thumb MCP	Flexion	0 - 50
	Extension	0
Thumb CMC	ABD	0 - 70
	ADD	0
	OPP	tip of thumb to tip or base of fifth digit
Wrist	Flexion	0 - 80
	Extension	0 - 70
	Radial Deviation	0 - 20
	Ulnar Deviation	0 - 30
	Pronation/Supination	0 - 90
Elbow	Flexion	0 - 150
	Extension	0 - 5
	Pronation/Supination	0 - 90
Shoulder	Flexion	0 - 180
	Extension	0 - 60
	ABD	0 - 180
	ADD	0 - 45
	Internal Rotation	0 - 70
	External Rotation	0 - 90
Hip	Flexion	0 - 120
	Extension	0 - 30
	ABD	0 - 45/50
	ADD	0 - 30
	Internal Rotation	0 - 35/45
	External Rotation	0 - 45
Knee	Flexion	0 - 135
	Extension	0
	Tibial Inversion	0 - 10
	Tibial Eversion	0 - 10
Ankle	Dorsiflexion	0 - 20
	Plantar Flexion	0 - 50
Subtalar	Inversion	0 - 5
	Eversion	0 - 5
Forefoot	Inversion	0 - 35
	Eversion	0 - 15
MTPs (Toes 2 - 5)	Flexion	0 - 40
	Extension	0 - 40
MTP (First Toe)	Flexion	0 - 45
	Extension	0 - 70
IP (First Toe)	Flexion	0 - 4
	Extension	0

Appendix 1.3

Synovial Fluid Analysis: The Three "C's"

Classification of Synovial Fluid	Cells (WBC/mm^3)	Crystal	Culture
Normal	< 200	Negative	Negative
Noninflammatory (e.g., osteoarthritis)	< 2000	Negative	Negative
Inflammatory	2000 - 100,000 and > 50% PMNs	Positive in Gout, CPPD Negative in autoimmune inflammatory arthropathies e.g., RA, SLE, Psoriatic Arthritis etc)	Negative
Septic	> 50,000 > 75% PMNs	May have rare calcium pyrophosphate crystal	Positive
Hemorragic	Not applicable (frank blood)	Negative	Negative

Appendix 1.4

Glossary

This is not meant to be a comprehensive list, but here are some frequently used words or phrases that sometimes give rise to confusion.

Anatomical Snuff Box. Area over the radial (thumb side) aspect of the wrist bounded by the extensor pollicus longus and extensor pollicus brevis tendons. The scaphoid bone forms the floor of the box.

Bouchard's nodes. Named after the physician who first described them. These are osteophytes at the proximal interphalangeal joints.

Boutonniere deformity. When swelling or trauma disrupt the volar plate of the PIP joint, the finger extensor tendons slip on either side of the PIP joint pulling the DIP joint into extension and the PIP joint into flexion. Picture the joint as a button being pulled through a button hole, hence the name.

Glossary (continued)

Carrying angle of the elbow. The angle of the upper arm in relation to the lower arm.

CMC joint. Capal metacarpal joint. The wrist attaches to the hand via these joints.

DIP joint. Distal interphalangeal joint of any digit (fingers or toes). These are the furthest or most distal joints in the hand or foot.

Heberden's nodes. Named after the physician who described them, they are identical to Bouchard's nodes except the osteophytes are at the DIP joints.

Mallet finger. The DIP joint of the finger is in flexion and cannot be actively extended. It is caused by loss of attachment of the extensor tendon at the DIP joint. This is a common injury, frequently seen in ball players.

MCP joint. Metacarpal phalangeal joint, in lay terms, the hand's knuckles. These joints attach the fingers to the hand. Their counterpart in the foot are the metatarsal phalangeal joints (MTP joints).

PIP joint. The proximal interphalangeal joint of any digit (fingers or toes). These are the joints between the distal interphalngeal joints and the joints that attach the digits to the hand or foot (MCP & MTP joints).

Pronation. Used in reference to the forearm, foot and body, it has the following meanings: 1) the movement of the forearm that allows the palm to face down, 2) the movement of the foot that brings the outer foot up, the medial foot down; it is a rotational force through the long axis of the foot, 3) the act of lying face down.

Radial. On the same side as, or movement toward, the forearm bone labelled the radius. The thumb is on the same side as the radius.

Supination. This word has two meanings: 1) the position of lying on the back and 2) the movement of the forearm that allows the palm to face up. In the absence of a cup or a bowl, this is the position you would try and hold water or soup (soupination) in your hand.

Swan Neck Deformity. Finger deformity characterized by flexion of the MCP joint, hyperextension of the PIP joint and flexion of the DIP joint of the same finger. It is a result of chronic inflammation in the MCP and PIP joints causing ligamentous stretch, and is frequently seen in rheumatoid arthritis and systemic lupus erythematosus.

Ulnar. On the same side as, or movement toward, the forearm bone labelled the ulna.

Valgus. The position of a joint when the distal limb is angled away from the midline of the body. Example: in the knee, valgus angulation of both knees results in 'knock knees'.

Varus. The position of a joint when the distal limb is angled toward the midline of the body. Example: in the knee, varus angulation of both knees results in 'bow legs', as if the patient had been riding a horse.

Appendix 1.5

References and Source Material

Textbooks

Dandy, David. Essential Orthopedics and Trauma, New York: Churchill Livingstone, 1989.

Doherty, Michael, Brian Hazleman, Charles Hutton, Peter Maddison, J David Perry. Rheumatology Examination and Injection Techniques. Toronto: W.B. Saunders Company Ltd., 1992.

Gross, Jeffrey, Joseph Fetto, Elaine Rosen. Musculoskeletal Examination Second Edition. Ames, Iowa: Blackwell Science, Inc., 2002.

Hoppenfeld, Stanley. Physical Examination of the Spine and Extremities. Norwalk, Conneticut, Appleton-Century-Crofts, 1976.

Magee, David. Orthopedic Physical Assessment. W.B. Saunders Company. Toronto, Ont. 1987.

Peer Reviewed Literature

Upper Extremity Assessment

Carmeli E, Patish H, Coleman R.The aging hand. J Gerontol A Biol Sci Med Sci. 2003 Feb;58(2):146-52.

Morgan WJ, Slowman LS. Acute hand and wrist injuries in athletes: evaluation and management. J Am Acad Orthop Surg. 2001 Nov-Dec;9(6):389-400.

Slater, RR, Jr. Carpal tunnel syndrome: current concepts. J South Orthop Assoc. 1999 Fall;8(3):203-13.

Kapandji, AI. The clinical evaluation of the upper limb joints' function: back to Hippocrates. Hand Clin. 2003 Aug;19(3):379-86.

Onieal ME. Common wrist and elbow injuries in primary care. Lippincotts Prim Care Pract. 1999 Jul-Aug;3(4):441-50.

Septic olecranon bursitis: recognition and treatment. J Am Board Fam Pract. 1995 May-Jun;8(3):217-20.

Meister, K. Injuries to the shoulder in the throwing athlete. Part one: Biomechanics/ pathophysiology/classification of injury. Am J Sports Med. 2000 Mar-Apr;28(2):265-75.

Spine Assessment

Honet JC, Ellenberg MR. What you always wanted to know about the history and physical examination of neck pain but were afraid to ask. Phys Med Rehabil Clin N Am. 2003 Aug; 14(3): 473-91.

Levy HI. Cervical pain syndromes: primary care diagnosis and management. Compr Ther. 2000 Summer; 26(2): 82-8.

Moskovich R. Neck pain in the elderly: common causes and management. Geriatrics. 1988 Apr; 43(4): 65-70, 77, 81-2 passim.

Rao R. Neck pain, cervical radiculopathy, and cervical myelopathy: pathophysiology, natural history, and clinical evaluation. Instr Course Lect. 2003; 52: 479-88

Thomas, SA Spinal stenosis: history and physical examination. Phys Med Rehabil Clin N Am. 2003 Feb;14(1):29-39.

Lower Extremity Assessment

DeAngelis,NA, Busconi, BD. Assessment and differential diagnosis of the painful hip.

Clin Orthop. 2003 Jan;(406): 11-8.

Zacher,J, Gursche,A. Regional musculoskeletal condition: 'hip' pain. Best Pract Res Clin Rheumatol. 2003 Feb; 17(1):71-85.

Murphy, PC, Knight AS. Misdiagnosis in sports medicine. Curr Sports Med Rep. 2002 Dec;1(6):333-7.

Keene, J Diagnosis of undetected knee injuries. Interpreting subtle clinical and radiologic findings. Postgrad Med. 1989 Mar;85(4):153-6, 161-3.

Lee TK, Maleski R. Physical examination of the ankle for ankle pathology. Clin Podiatr Med Surg. 2002 Apr;19(2):251-69.

Swain,RA, Holt, W.S. Ankle injuries. Tips from sports medicine physicians.Postgrad Med. 1993 Feb 15; 93(3): 91-2, 97-100.

Balint GP, Korda J, Hangody L, Balint PV. Regional musculoskeletal conditions: foot and ankle disorders. Best Pract Res Clin Rheumatol. 2003 Feb; 17(1): 87-111

Chambers HG, Sutherland DH. A practical guide to gait analysis. Am Acad Orthop Surg. 2002 May-Jun;10(3):222-31.

Hockenbury RT. Forefoot problems in athletes. Med Sci Sports Exerc. 1999 Jul;31(7 Suppl): S448-58.

Kravitz SR, McGuire J, Shanahan SD. Physical assessment of the diabetic foot. Adv Skin Wound Care. 2003 Mar-Apr;16(2):68-75; quiz A022-3.

Screening Examination

Doherty M, Dacre J, Dieppe P, Snaith M. The 'GALS' locomotor screen. Ann Rheum Dis 1992;51(10):1165-9.

Foster HE, Kay LJ, Friswell M, Coady D, Myers A. Musculoskeletal screening examination (pGALS) for school-age children based on the adult GALS screen. Arthritis Rheum 2006;55(5):709-16.

Fox RA, Dacre JE, Clark CL, Scotland AD. Impact on medical students of incorporating GALS screen teaching into the medical school curriculum. Ann Rheum Dis 2000;59(9):668-71.

Lillicrap MS, Byrne E, Speed CA. Musculoskeletal assessment of general medical in-patients--joints still crying out for attention. Rheumatology (Oxford) 2003;42(8):951-4.

Plant MJ, Linton S, Dodd E, Jones PW, Dawes PT. The GALS locomotor screen and disability. Ann Rheum Dis 1993;52(12):886-90.

ABOUT THE AUTHOR

Dr. Sutton is Professor of Medicine and Head, Division of Rheumatology in Dalhousie University's Department of Medicine in Halifax, Nova Scotia, Canada. She is also Director of the Arthritis Center of Nova Scotia. She has received numerous teaching awards, including the 2006 Canadian Association of Medical Education's Certificate of Merit and Dalhousie's Department of Medicine Excellence in Education award. She is an active member of several professional associations and speaks frequently as an invited lecturer.